Healthy Body, Healthy Mind,
Healthy Life

Part II

Nutrition For Exercise

JOE BOONE

CSCS, CISSN

COPYRIGHT & DISCLAIMER

TABLE OF CONTENTS

INTRODUCTION

In *Healthy Body, Healthy Mind, Healthy Life Part II: Nutrition for Exercise* we look at the many aspects that surround giving the body nutrients for training and performance, including supplementation. These topics are important. When a specific goal has been established the methods have to become more specific. Feeding the exercise and fueling the muscle are crucial when exercise is part of the process.

Just like in nutrition outside of the exercise context people sensationalize ideas and the big picture loses its value. Claims come about and its the only way that will work and all others are inferior. You have to understand the basics in order for any of these claims to even be considered as options. There will always be dietary methods being pushed as an attempt at enhancing goals like fat loss, mass gain, performance, etc in the context of exercise, but too many times people forget that nutrition is only one piece of the puzzle and it is there to fuel the training. Food doesn't make you loose weight. Food doesn't make you gain weight. Food should not be the focus. Your focus should be on your training. The food is simply added in to the equation to optimize goal attainment.

The concepts covered in *Healthy Body, Healthy Mind, Healthy Life Part I: Nutrition* provide a good base of knowledge to work off of. Understanding the foundational information can aid you in attaining whatever your goal is without being sucked into the pseudo-science and people's belief systems that surround how they eat. When nutrition is applied to training it should be based on the same as outside of exercise -- the evidence, your goals, what you like, and trial and error. Although with training in the picture it becomes more complex.

I hope that what I have given you in the following text provides some clarity to the complex issue. I think having a grasp on the dynamics of this topic and some of the evidence really allows optimization of any goal. Nutrition is simple yet complicated and is a big part of daily life, understanding it really takes some pressure off of the process.

In this text there is science communicated via citations. It is important to understand that all research reports means, or the averages, of the results. That means that these concepts should be taken as a general construct to assist in your journey, as some results are higher than the reported average and some are lower. This is not the only downfall to research. There are many limitations, and there is no such thing as a perfect study, especially when humans are the subjects. We humans have a life to live and can't be studied in an isolated environment the way some other species and cells can. Understand that the results of research provides information that is applicable to your life, and being able to use it to your advantage is the most important thing to take away. It should not be viewed as law.

I hope you enjoy Part II of the four part series of *Healthy Body, Healthy Mind, Healthy Life.*

-Joe Boone

1 WELLNESS, THE CENTER OF PROGRESSION

HEALTH, FITNESS, AND WELLNESS DEFINED

Health may be defined as the absence of disease or a diseased state. According to this definition, when you hear someone say they want to become "healthier," they are, in a sense, admitting their current lifestyle decisions are not optimal. Whether it is eating processed food, fast food, excess food, getting too little exercise, or other harmful behaviors, these actions keep us from living a healthy lifestyle [1 – 3]. This is health as it is related to the physical body.

The term "health" may be further broken down into subcomponents, including mental and social aspects. Being healthy is not just the absence of disease in the body. It is also the well-being of the mind and an individual's psychosocial life, or the relationships a person has with other people. These three things are tightly woven together, and this chapter will bring some light to how integral their relationship is.

There is a fourth aspect to a person's health that goes deeper than what the eye can see, and that is spiritual health. The physical, mental, and social subcomponents are manifestations of the physical health of the body and its parts. The mind is made up of physical organs and social relationships are made of people, and all of these things are tangible parts of life. Unlike these aspects of health, the spiritual component is not as easy to see, but it's equally important. Spirituality and spiritual health generally mean having a sense of meaning or purpose and a connection to a set of values which guide that purpose. How you establish spiritual health and your spirituality is dependent on your belief systems.

Spirituality has a big impact on your life. Are you able to understand the meaning of the things that happen? Are you able to accept there are things you cannot change? Your spiritualty has a huge impact on your mental health. If your perception does not allow you to accept what is happening around you, then your mindset is altered, and that is what determines your mental and ultimately even your emotional health.

Fitness can be defined as a measurable level of ability. Generally, in biology, an organism's fitness level is judged by whether or not it can reproduce and survive its environment [4]. Is the organism fit enough to pass on its genetic material? The popular slogan "survival of the fittest" says it all. In physical fitness this translates to many things one being reduction of disease risk, which allows a person to live a longer and healthier life. For example, level of fitness has a direct relationship to risk of early death [5], the more fit the less likely to die early. That results in the ability of a fit person to live a longer and potentially more enjoyable life than someone who is less fit.

Wellness is defined as a general sense of well-being. Simply, it is the compilation of health and fitness-- the absence of disease, a highly functioning mind, relationships that are mutually beneficial, and in a general sense a high level of functioning in your body and across life. Are there some limitations to that? Yes, but we can all strive to improve our individual levels by first understanding what they mean.

How They are Related

Defining and differentiating between health, fitness, and wellness helps us understand how they are all different. But it also helps us understand how they are linked to each other. Let's take a look at their relationship. Do you specifically know how your level of health is tied to your fitness and wellness?

Under all three terms there are many components. These include emotional, mental, relational, social, muscular, cardiovascular, and financial. The list could go on, but the fact is that the components of health, fitness, and wellness all come together and shape how you live your life.

The healthier you are the greater potential you have to function at a higher output in the tangible and intangible portions of your life. It may be variable from person to person, but overall the more fit you are physically, mentally, socially, and spiritually, the greater potential there is for improved quality of wellness across life as a spectrum. Health manifests in so many other ways that influence your quality of life, which is why health and wealth have a relationship. Health often correlates with fitness [5], and therefore wellness. The more well you are the greater your potential to excel in other areas of your life. Is wealth necessarily tied to the amount of zeros in your bank account? No, there is much more to wealth.

Wealth is subjective to what your goals in life are, and it is up to you to decide what makes you wealthy. Is it having a large family with people that support and love each other? Is it accomplishing personal career goals? Is it having a small group of friends to call on when you need them the most? Is it being educated? Is it financial wealth? This is something you must decide for yourself. The work you have to do to reach those goals will depend on your overall health and fitness.

The likelihood of you being able to perform at the top of your game and be wealthy is not high if your body is burdened with disease. Success is not likely if you're on the lower echelons of physical capability, or your general sense of being is negative. How can you have a high output on pursing a goal if your emotional state is out of whack? How can you achieve a wealthy life, whatever that means to you, if you look at the world in a negative light? How can you achieve what you want to achieve without generally being well?

It is not impossible, but the more healthy you are, the more fit you are likely to be and the more likely you are to have a higher sense of well-being. This manifests all across your life.

Understanding how to get there is a very dynamic and ever-changing path, so it is important to understand that the psychological aspect may be the hardest part. Can you use that mind of yours to evaluate what needs to be evaluated and accept what needs to be accepted? Motivation, psychology and mindset are highly intertwined and have a relationship comparable to that of the molecules that make up our cells. Your ability to develop your mindset and know that there will be failures is crucial; you have to be able to pick yourself up and learn from every experience. After all, failure is just another word for lesson. The people that you view as successful did not make it to the place they are in life without stumbling down the path and being beaten up by its obstacles. They took the beating, got back up, and continued on stronger.

Obviously, health and wellness are linked together. But to reach our goals and fully understand each aspect, we must break it down into the specific components. In *Healthy Body, Healthy Mind, Healthy Life Part II: Nutrition for Exercise* we look at the aspects of the diet in relation to training on the path to a more well self.

EXERCISE FOR NUTRITION

For anyone with specific goals, whether they are weight loss or gain, health, performance or some combination, nutrition is an integral part of the process. Understanding the relationship between the body and nutrition is essential to reaching any health or performance goal. The benefits of understanding these concepts are not limited to those discussed in *Healthy Body, Healthy Mind, Healthy Life Part I: Nutrition*. This book provides more knowledge on the topics related to reaching gym related goals in the attempt to allow you to build yourself from the nutritional perspective.

2   WHEN AND HOW OFTEN TO EAT

The general nutritional suggestions from Part I of *Healthy Body, Healthy Mind, Healthy Life (Nutrition)* include eating the appropriate portions according to your energy needs, limiting or excluding processed and fried foods, and eating enough protein and fiber. Limiting your palate makes it difficult to meet these suggestions. Yes, vegetarian and other dietary variations do have benefits, but a balanced and adequate nutrient intake comes from eating from all food groups.

Knowing when and how often to eat is the next step, but these things are not concrete across the board because you must always consider your individual characteristics. The most significant barrier seems to be schedule and convenience when it comes to nutritional intake and exercise. Even with the challenges, if the goals are worth it you will find a way to make it happen.

The first thing to understand is that the body's primary fuel comes from the breakdown of glucose. Glucose is maintained at certain levels in an acceptable range in blood for the tissues that use it, primarily the skeletal muscle and nervous system. The nervous system always supersedes the skeletal muscle in glucose provided from blood because muscle cells contain their own personal stores called glycogen.

Long periods without eating causes blood sugar to be reduced. The body only stores a limited amount of glucose to maintain blood levels. For the purposes of blood sugar maintenance, the body uses liver stores where there are roughly eight hours' worth. As you sleep or go through a period of not eating (fasting) these stores are used to maintain the blood sugar. They can become depleted to a degree which has an impact on the dynamics of hunger and even fatigue and mood state (have you ever experienced hanger?). It is variable, but partially why some people are hungry as soon as they wake up.

If you do not eat upon waking you extend this period of fasting beyond those eight hours, and the pathways that result in protein breakdown become more active [6]. This is where proteins are used to create new glucose at a higher rate than they normally would in the presence of a meal. The body is in a constant cycle of building up and breaking down. Extended periods of fasting causes the amount of breakdown to outweigh the amount of building. In the fasted state there is also an increased ability for active tissue to use fat as a fuel [7,8]. But breaking down protein at a greater rate than it is built does not have positive implications for those that are trying to achieve any positive goal.

There are two general types of biological processes, catabolic and anabolic, breaking down and building up. They are usually coupled, so when a catabolic or breakdown reaction occurs, an anabolic or building reaction will follow. In the case of fat or protein catabolism, breakdown will produce biological components that can be used to build new glucose molecules.

In a fasted state, protein and fats are used more for energy than they would be in a fed state. This is usually because your carbohydrate stores are low, or lower than your body likes them to be. When fat is broken down, the fatty acids are removed from their backbone, the glycerol. Both the fatty acids and the glycerol can be used for energy production, or in some manner. Increased fat catabolism is a huge factor for those with a fat loss goal, but most people seem to forget that in order for this to matter you have to create a caloric deficit to have a positive change in body fat. It's not just about increasing fat breakdown. It is about providing the nutritional and exercise conditions that facilitate this positive change.

Fasting is a newer area of research, but it seems that the intermittent fast protocol (where there are specific feeding and fasting periods) is an effective dietary program for fat loss. The research suggests that with resistance exercise, strength and lean mass can be maintained while fat and overall mass are lost [9]. However, it should be noted that the intermittent fast may not provide the conditions necessary for optimizing any type of performance adaptation. In short, fasting can be used but it is best applied when the goal is weight loss.

Ingesting any calories sends a signal for the body to release insulin, and insulin tells the cells to take in and use carbohydrates. When insulin levels are high carbohydrate becomes the priority; the breakdown of fat and protein are slowed. When insulin levels are lower, the protein and fat energy pathways or what can be called faucets are 'turned up'. This is why the timing of your food intake can be important. Depending on your goals and health status, you will want to eat either more frequently or less frequently. When you eat less frequently your meals will have to be larger. This ensures the energy intake is met even though there are less opportunities to get all of your calories in. This is also where meal preparation becomes significant, as having those meals ready to go when you need them is crucial for convenience.

Meal preparation is especially significant in a nutritional program that allows for more frequent feeding times. You will want those meals ready to go so they do not interfere with the rest of your schedule. In regards to one or the other, you will have to choose which works best for your goals and life. One of the most important things to keep in the back of your head is that eating is a part of your lifestyle. Whatever you do, it must be something that you enjoy and can maintain.

When it comes to the differences between frequent and infrequent eating, there is some science to be considered. To start, there is an idea that frequent eating increases your metabolism. That is not actually true, in fact, it lowers resting metabolism. The scientific literature suggests that increasing meal frequency does not increase resting metabolism or improve body composition [10]. However, in the presence of adequate protein intake, more frequent eating can help maintain lean mass when in a caloric deficit [10].

Since we have put the myth about meal frequency and metabolism to rest, we also need to bring light to the other truths of increased meal frequency. Eating frequently may improve blood markers, decrease hunger, and improve appetite control [11]. We must take these things in consideration but try not to get hung up on every piece of evidence.

When it comes to infrequent eating, there are also ideas that need to be cleared up. Most recently, intermittent fasts have become popular. We will tie these ideas to the research performed with that style of nutritional manipulation. One theory that disputes infrequent eating is that putting the body into a starvation state causes the storage of extra fat. We already discovered there is research that shows the body is actually burning more fat and is capable of using fat more readily in the fasted state, so that idea needs to be put to rest, but it cannot be forgotten that catabolism does become greater with less feeding. This is somewhat tied to the fewer feeding opportunities, meaning less insulin is being released and more reliance on local energy stores. A reduced amount of feeding times in the day has also been shown to be promising for improving health markers, reducing total body weight, and reducing body fat, which may be especially significant to overweight and overfat populations [12, 13].

An infrequent feeding plan requires the individual to get all daily calories in fewer meals [9] and may help when the goal is to decrease the total amount of calories taken in per day. This is significant especially for those trying to create an energy deficit to make fat loss efficient. It may even create conditions that allow for an energy deficit without even knowing it is happening.

When it comes to the frequency of eating, the research seems to support both infrequent (less than three meals per day) and frequent (more than three meals per day). A person's goals determine which plan is best. If your goal is extreme weight loss and the improvement of health markers, it seems more beneficial to use the intermittent fast that includes those fewer feeding times. If you are trying to build lean mass, fewer eating periods will likely not help you attain your goal and you may want to shoot for more than three times per day. The one thing that must not be forgotten is that dietary protein helps stimulate protein synthesis in the constant process of whole body protein turnover. This battle between anabolism and catabolism rotates back and forth approximately every three hours if the appropriate stimulus is met. This three hour period is called the protein synthesis refractory period and why it is optimal to ingest adequate protein about every three hours.

What about the typical three meals per day? Well, once again, your nutrition must be driven by your goal. For a goal of maintenance and appetite control, the research seems to show that the standard three times per day may actually be the best option [11].

It is obvious your goal is what will determine how frequently you will eat. But there are also other considerations to make, including what you enjoy and if it works with your schedule. When you are going after goals you must be able to adapt your methods to find the best way for *you* to reach them. Even when research and trends are touting one specific way, you might find that way doesn't work at all for you. If that is the case you must be able to take it as a learning experience and try again with another method. I find that the best methods are often combinations of what most people consider good plans.

Reaching goals tied to nutritional intake cannot be viewed as short-term. You eat multiple times every day, so you must also look at the long-term and how today will impact tomorrow and years from now. After all, it is your life you are trying to make a difference with, not just one meal.

3 FUELING EXERCISE AND FEEDING THE MUSCLE

When you apply an eating plan to exercise it becomes a little more complicated and more specific than just eating to maintain a healthy lifestyle. Now you have to consider eating as fuel for your exercise as well as timing your eating for optimum results.

PRE-WORKOUT FUEL

The idea behind the pre-workout snack is to increase the fuel your muscles have access to during an exercise session. When planning a pre-workout snack, think about the fuel your body uses during exercise. Generally, the more intense the workout, the more carbohydrates are used, and the less intense the workout, the more fats are used. The longer you exercise, the more fat is burned and the shorter the exercise the more carbohydrate is burned [14]. Protein, in most cases, only provides about five percent of the calories used during a workout, but it can provide up to ten percent [15] if it is an extended bout where the other fuels are being depleted to levels lower than the body is comfortable with. No matter what fuel is dominant in exercise metabolism, we must not forget the concept of the fuel faucets; where carbohydrate, fat, and protein each have their own faucet that is always on. In addition to the faucets, the majority of the fuels that are being used during exercise are coming from stores already in the body, not those ingested. Pre-workout snacks can be effective, but in many cases they may not be required.

If you pay attention to the fuel that is used and its relationship to duration and intensity, that will tell you a lot about what you should eat. In fact, duration and intensity are two very significant factors that you will need to continue to pay attention to. In regards to fuel, the muscle stores local carbohydrate as glycogen, and it also has local stores of fat. As a back-up there are stores of carbohydrate in the liver. If you are eating in a normal pattern and not extending fast periods, these stores will be able to supply your exercise with the fuel it needs. The body is capable of supplying its muscles with energy without a specific snack. But if your workouts are excessively long and/or intense, then the stores can start to become relatively depleted to levels that the body is uncomfortable with. At these times, ingestion of energy may be beneficial for performance.

Knowing what we know about intensity, duration, and fuel sources, we can see how the different modes will use predominantly different fuels. Resistance training, or workouts that are generally more anaerobic, will mostly rely on carbohydrates, while endurance training, or workouts that are generally more aerobic, will rely predominantly on fat (but this is very dependent on the intensity/duration). That does not mean that those are exclusively the fuels, but when we look at fueling the workout these are important to consider.

When it comes to fat as a fuel, typically there is already a lot stored. This is because the body likes to hold on to excess energy, and we can store an unlimited amount of energy in fat. The glucose in the blood is mainly there to fuel the brain, so the muscles rely on their own stores of glycogen. You may have heard the term glycogen depletion from a person talking about their resistance training. They were correct in recognizing that their muscles were using those stores of carbohydrates, but depletion is a relative term. The limited research that has evaluated glycogen depletion and resistance training suggests that there is only about thirty-five percent depletion of the local glycogen [16]. Though research finds this is the case, it may be possible to deplete further than this; it all depends on duration and intensity.

The body's first goal is preservation to ensure survival (carbohydrate is a quick and easy fuel), so when glycogen is depleted even by thirty-five percent or less it will begin to switch to other fuels, which will impair performance. In this instance it could be beneficial to ingest a carbohydrate food that would increase the blood concentration of carbohydrate for the muscles to take from.

The key take away is that it is the intensity and duration that matter most. If you deplete fuel stores, the body begins to adjust what fuel is used at what rate, and that can impact performance. Runners experience this when they hit "the wall." Considering the longer the exercise the more it becomes anaerobic, supplementing a workout with an easily digestible carbohydrate can be beneficial in those very long and intense bouts.

AFTER THE WORKOUT

You must always remember that the biological programming of the body is to maintain life and the conditions that allow life to happen. Essentially, the body always thinks it is going to die.

First, when the term glycogen depletion is heard it sounds as if all glycogen is gone, but in reality it is relative depletion. That being the case, it may not be necessary to load your muscles with a ridiculous amount of carbs in that post-workout meal. Research shows that without carbohydrate ingestion the body will still resynthesize its lost glycogen [17]. This is tied to that biological programming of maintaining the conditions that allow life to be sustained. Specifically, having a supply of local fuel in case there is a life-threatening situation where the muscle will be required to contract as a reaction. Therefore, immediate carbohydrate intake is not a necessity to replenish any glycogen that is depleted, but in cases it can be advantageous.

When talking about muscle, we are talking about a tissue that is able to produce movement through the action of contractile proteins. Those proteins receive damage, and the inherent goal of exercise is to build more efficient and productive muscle while we are actually purposely breaking it down. With your new understanding of whole body turnover and the knowledge that the exercising muscle receives damage, you know that you have to supply the body with enough protein and amino acids to ensure you can actually achieve the goal of creating more total body protein. We know this is not an easy goal. So what is the right way to fuel the muscle with protein?

We have learned the dynamics of different feeding times and how it affects anabolism and catabolism, but how does exercise play into all of this? Protein intake benefits all types of exercise because it is needed for optimal synthesis. In fact, research suggests that ingesting protein before a workout is more beneficial for increasing protein synthesis when compared to ingesting after [18]. This may be due to the increased amino acid availability for the muscle during the exercise, which reduces the catabolic effect of exercise, allowing for greater potential to build more muscle once the workout is complete. This does not mean that protein intake following exercise is inefficient, it actually means that there is benefit to both. There are studies suggesting that protein synthesis is improved and enhanced by both the pre- and post-exercise protein intake [18], as long as there is protein intake in proximity to the exercise session. Really, it comes down to you and the specifics of your training.

When it comes to post exercise intake, people often refer to certain windows of time. The anabolic window represents the thirty minute to one hour period immediately following a workout where protein synthesis has been claimed to be at its peak. There is also the three hour period following an exercise where there is increased muscle protein synthesis [18]. There is even recent research that has explored the anabolic effect on muscle extending into the four to six hour post exercise timeframe [19]. This indicates that exercise itself is anabolic, and protein intake is supplemental to that affect, optimizing it as much as six hours after. That means as long as you are eating protein at some point after the exercise you will be increasing protein synthesis. That thirty minute window is great if you like the immediate post intake, but it is not crucial if you are not hungry. In determining how long you want to wait, it must be considered that the longer you wait, the less time during the day you have to ingest the total amount of protein you need to be in a positive state of protein building. It is possible to wait and still receive benefits, but it may not be conducive to increasing total lean mass in the long term, one meal does not meet your daily requirement.

Due to the protein synthetic refractory period, the battle of increasing whole body protein, and the anabolic stimulus that protein and the amino acid intake cause [20], it is common to see people who resistance train eat a protein food source every three hours. This ensures they are setting optimal conditions for accomplishing the goal of positive gain in muscle mass. However, do not forget that there is leeway on that three hour period and post exercise ingestion, because exercise itself is anabolic. Instead of the anabolic window it should be called the anabolic door-way.

Exercise isn't the only factor in considering what times of day to eat. You may have heard that eating after a certain hour will cause you to store more fat, but is that really true? And how does the recommendation not to eat late in the evening affect the pre-bedtime protein shake, or eating to fulfill your caloric needs?

We set daily caloric needs for important reasons, all based around the individual. Those needs have to be met to facilitate the desired outcome. If at the end of the day you have not met your needs, then it is important that you do that, especially if the goal has something to do with body composition or performance. The message that has been expressed saying that it is bad to eat after a certain hour because of a mysterious fat storing quality of a time of day is incorrect. It is not true that eating later will cause you to store more fat. The reality is that our cravings for a snack are not always healthy and have the potential of adding calories into our intake that we do not need.

Food selection and snacking can easily become mindless activity that can take you over your energy goal for the day. If you are able to choose a snack or food that falls into your plan and you have the self-control to limit the intake, then eating late does not matter. However, if you don't control the factors then they will control the outcome. According to a research review on this topic, what seems to be a better predictor of weight gain and the association to sleep is having shorter sleeping cycles [21]. This allows for a longer waking period and therefore more waking time in the day for intake of total calories. Simply put, if you are awake for more hours during a twenty-four hour period you might eat more.

When it comes to eating, understanding that there are over four thousand processes that occur in trillions of cells is crucial. Each person has their own individual energy production, and applying the individual factor to those four thousand processes is critical to understanding that your body is not a cookie cutter. It is key to understanding that some styles of dietary intake will not work for you, while others will. This is why knowing your body and being able to change things when something is not working is key. You have to be fluid with your journey and have fun with it. You should also have all of the facts so that you are prepared to attack your goals and have the tools you need to succeed. One of those tools is understanding just how important your dietary intake actually is. This includes understanding how all four macronutrients, especially protein, work in the presence of exercise. You must not forget the functions of the macronutrients and what your body is going to do with them.

A DEEPER LOOK AT PROTEIN

Carbohydrates and fats have the primary role of fuel in relation to the different intensities and metabolic pathways. They both have other functions as well, but their primary role is in fueling and driving cellular activity through their breakdown into molecules that are then put together to form ATP (Adenosine Triphosphate) molecule. ATP is coined biological energy currency and what your food is transformed into so that your body can use it to fuel its cells. The bottom line is that carbohydrates and fats are broken down so that the cells may make ATP and drive all cellular activity out of that ATP. This is important because our cellular activity is what keeps us going, and protein is an important part of this equation.

Let's not forget there is a nucleus in each cell and the processes that are driven by the cell and the nucleus are all fueled by ATP. The primary function of the nucleus is to provide instructions for building new proteins. The nucleus of the many cells drive protein synthesis (not just in muscle) to create the thousands of proteins that DNA tells it to. This is why the body does not like to use dietary protein as fuel, and why getting enough protein in the diet is so important. The many functions that come out of these play roles in growth and maintenance, hormonal, biological catalysts (enzymes), antibodies (immune function), pH (acid-base) balance, fluid and water balance, and transportation of components through the body.

Proteins are found in a variety of sources. It is difficult but possible to get the right amount of amino acids from a plant-based diet by combining different foods with the complementation of amino acids. In doing this the sources complete each other in regards to the amino acid availability.

The RDA of protein is set at 0.8 grams of protein for every kilogram of bodyweight per day [22]. This recommendation is based on sedentary activity levels and trying to prevent deficiency. Anyone who is more than sedentary will require a greater amount than 0.8g of dietary protein per kilogram of body weight daily, and really sedentary individuals should be ingesting more than the minimum. We have to remember that whole body protein turnover is occurring on a regular basis no matter the activity level, so supplying new sources for the body to maintain what is there is crucial. Increasing the amount of activity only increases the need for dietary protein.

Let's take a 150 pound person as an example on the protein RDA. To convert to kilograms we divide 150 by 2.2, and that puts that person at about 68.2 kilograms. To determine what they need to be eating to meet the RDA, multiply 68.2 by 0.8g. That gives us 54.6 grams. For that person to meet the RDA for protein they would only have to eat about 55 grams of protein in a day. To see what that equates to in calories we multiply 55 by 4, since that is how many calories there are in a gram of protein. That gives us 220 calories per day from protein. Using the generic 2000 calorie model we can see how that is not very significant, in fact it only comes to about 11 percent of the 2,000 calories. That means the other 89 percent has to come from carbohydrates and fat. That may not be an issue, however, it is still a *very low* amount of protein.

If you are an exercising individual you will need more than 0.8g of protein per kilogram. In fact, research supports a range that is nearly double that at 1.4 – 2.0g of protein per kilogram of body weight for healthy adults that regularly participate in structured exercise [23]. The type of exercise will determine where on that scale is best, but in general it seems the more resistance training, the higher the requirement for dietary protein. If we are to use that same 150 pound (68.2 kilogram) person, even at 1.7g per kilogram, in the middle of the range, it more than doubles the RDA, putting the daily grams of protein intake to 116, which is 464 calories and now 23 percent of the 2,000 calorie diet. That is a huge difference and will have a significant impact of the body's ability to maintain and build body tissues, not just muscle, and provide many other benefits.

Protein intake is an area of constant research in the sports nutrition realm, but protein is not just applicable to performance. It is important for all populations, from pediatrics to geriatrics, from elite athletes to the different clinical populations. You must not forget that it is not just your skeletal muscles that are made of proteins and amino acids; even tissues like your bones and nervous system have significant protein content.

There are many benefits that dietary protein provides, but on the other side there is a negative light to protein intake and its impact on the body's general health. This negative is in how high protein intake influences hydration status, heart, kidney, liver, and bone health.

A major component of the protein molecule is nitrogen. The amino acid is named with amino or amine, because amine translates to nitrogen containing. The nitrogen content of protein was once thought to cause negative impacts on the body, such as increasing risk for cardiovascular disease, kidney and liver damage, and even decreasing bone density; but the research hasn't shown these things true in healthy people.

In one study that looked at protein, fat, and carbohydrate intake found that in comparison to a high carbohydrate diet group, a group that ate more protein and fat had a greater reduction in risk from cardiovascular disease and its blood markers. The group that was subjected to higher protein had greater positive changes in blood pressure, cholesterol, and triglycerides [24].

With the higher nitrogen intake, the primary concern has seemed to focus around the health and function of the kidneys and liver. These are the organs that function to filter blood, and because of that they are the organs that handle that extra nitrogen and rid the body of it.

When it comes to high protein intake, there have been no negative effects found in individuals with normal kidney function [25]. This specific research also indicates that the individuals that consumed a high-protein diet had no negative impacts on their excretion of other components like creatinine, albumin, and calcium. These things were originally thought to be why high-protein diets caused damage to the kidneys. Another interesting find was that the high protein intake resulted in a positive nitrogen balance, which is a key indicator for the relationship between whole body protein turnover and whether or not someone is consuming enough to battle protein breakdown.

Another concern in high-protein diets is calcium excretion. It used to be thought that the higher the intake of protein, the more calcium was pulled out of the bone. Research has shown this is not true. Research actually suggests a positive relationship between protein in the diet and bone health [26 – 28]. This positive relationship has even gone so far as to show that adequate protein in the diet decreases losses in bone mineral in premenopausal and perimenopausal women and increases bone mineral density in developing children when also consuming adequate calcium. Basically, you need adequate protein and calcium together in your diet to build and maintain strong bones.

Out of the negative relationships that were once tied to high protein in the diet the only one that seems to hold any merit is hydration status. Protein does require water for the body to process the excess nitrogen, and with that being the case there is more water excreted in urine. Ensuring proper hydration is important to all populations, but depending on the many individual factors, including protein intake, it can become a more important consideration. Loss of water can have a huge impact on performance and fatigue in exercise; if severe enough it can result in heat injuries.

A clearer picture of how protein works in the body allows us to understand that a greater amount of our caloric intake can and should come from protein. Some research has even looked at intake levels as high at 4.4 grams per kilogram per day [29]. The different ranges that have been studied are the RDA (0.8), 1.2-2.0, 1.3-1.6, 1.6-1.7, 1.4-2.0, 2.6-3.3, 3.4, and 4.4g/kg per day [23, 29, 30, 32, 34, 35]. As you can see, many ranges of protein intake have been researched to see the different impacts on the body and to learn what is optimal for who.

The research is clear in stating that even 3.4 grams per kilogram of body weight is safe and does not provide evidence of any deleterious effects on health [30, 32]. To put that into perspective, that is 4.25 times more than the RDA. Just to be clear, the study that looked at 4.4g/kg did not look at health markers, so we cannot say if that amount provides the same result. That study specially looked at a calorie surplus in resistance training males with that amount of protein, and there was *not* an increase in the participants' body fat [29]. This provides more support to the other topics we have discovered, and could be linked to that positive impact protein has on the thermal effect of feeding ((TEF, increased metabolism as a result of eating) [31, 33]. So, when it comes to protein intake, it is clear more isn't as bad as sometimes communicated.

The recommended amount for the active, exercising adult is 1.4 – 2.0g per kilogram of body weight per day [23]. That recommendation is made based on the research that has been done studying the adaptations received from exercise in conjunction with the intake of different amounts of protein. When looking at resistance training versus endurance training, the recommended protein intake will fall on different points in that 1.4 – 2.0g range. Resistance will be closer to the top and endurance a little lower than that. Mainly this is because resistance training is known to cause more damage and can require more dietary intake to ensure the threshold is met to allow for the building of a greater amount of skeletal muscle. Additionally, individuals that train endurance based exercise usually require greater amount of energy from fat and carbohydrate to ensure performance. There are some individuals that may fall outside of this range depending on the exercise stimulus and other factors, but meeting the 1.4 – 2.0g of protein per kilogram of bodyweight generally will provide the amount of protein needed.

The reason we recognize the 1.4 – 2.0 range as optimal is because the next range of 2.6 – 3.3 does not seem provide any additional benefits to performance or allow for significant increase in muscles mass [32]. *That is considered along with the fact that exercising individuals will still need to be able to fit the appropriate amounts of fat and carbohydrate in their intake to meet fuel requirements.* The 1.4 – 2.0g/kg/day range is recommended because we also now know that this level of intake is not detrimental to healthy people.

4 SUPPLEMENTATION, FROM PROBIOTIC TO ANABOLIC

When you hear the word supplementation or supplements, what is the first thing that comes to mind? For most people it is a body builder or someone who fits that stereotype. But supplementation has much more variation than that.

Supplementation is the scientific application of nutrients and biological agents to all populations in the pursuit of many diverse goals. These goals range from increasing performance to maintaining life with adequate nutritional intake. Supplementation to ensure proper nutrition in someone who has dietary restrictions or who cannot extract nutrients from certain foods is just one example, and one that is far different from a body builder slamming a post-workout shake to maximize gains during the "anabolic doorway." As you can see, there is potential for a wide variety of applications for supplementation. No matter what the reason for supplements, it is important to know the ingredients in the product, and what works and doesn't work.

The most common application of supplementing nutrition is in relation to exercise and performance.

The supplement market is a multibillion dollar industry, and there are a multitude of companies promoting products. When you drink a shake, eat a bar, or take a pill, do you actually know what that supplement is doing in your body, and does it really help get closer to reaching your goals?

THE MULTIVITAMIN MULTIMINERAL (MVMM)

The different vitamins and minerals are an important part of dietary intake. One of the first things to consider is your food selection. Are you eating a variety of foods, or are you someone who restricts your intake? If you restrict your diet there is a possibility you are limiting your micronutrient intake. For example, vegetarians do not eat meat, and meat not only contains the complete proteins and vitamin B12, but it is also rich in iron. In a research review iron deficiency was found to be the most common type of nutrient deficiency, estimated to impact more than 500 million people worldwide [36]. It is especially common in women of childbearing age due to menses and the resulting blood loss. Since iron is so significant in the cardiovascular system's ability to deliver oxygen, it is crucial that you get enough in the diet. The samples of the population that were taken give us an idea of how widespread this nutrient deficiency is and provides us with data to allow us to approach this issue and begin its resolution.

A diet that is not rich in iron can increase a person's risk of becoming deficient, especially in today's world where processed foods are often consumed. On the other side, we are seeing more foods fortified with iron and other nutrients. This does not necessarily mean you are meeting your need for iron, but it could be helping you get there. A diet low in iron can be associated with iron-deficiency anemia. This is the manifestation of low iron through low red blood cells, which leads to compromised ability to deliver oxygen and blood.

Another important nutrient is vitamin D. Since this fat-soluble vitamin has a strong relationship with calcium, the two are usually studied together. A deficiency in this vitamin has been shown to increase risk for decreases in bone mineral density as well as increase risk for metabolic conditions like Type-II diabetes [37 – 39]. In fact, supplementation of vitamin D and adequate calcium have even been found to decrease the rise in certain blood markers that are a result of Type-II diabetes and improve health of the pancreas [40].

Vitamin D has also been found to be beneficial in exercise-related supplementation due to its impact on calcium [41]. Calcium is a significant component of bone mineral composition, but it also plays a very important role in the contractile process of muscle cells. Supplementation of vitamin D seems to have a role in increasing muscular function via the action of increasing the capacity of muscle to use calcium. Interestingly, a review of the research that has investigated the supplementation of vitamin D by itself resulted in no significant benefit to bone mineral density [42]. This review allows us to look at vitamin D and its relationship with calcium. Since impacts to bone mineral density are not seen if calcium is not adequate, we can posit that the same is true with muscular function. This is because ninety-nine percent of the body's calcium is stored in the skeletal system; the remainder is allotted to muscular function and the other roles. In order to receive a benefit there must be adequate calcium intake in conjunction with vitamin D. This is a truth that applies broadly across other nutrients as well; different nutrients have different relationships to each other and the combinations affect how the body will be able to use them.

Iron and vitamin D are not the only micronutrients that are easily missed in the diet. If you are not getting the full range of micronutrients in the amounts you need you may want to consider the Multivitamin Multimineral (MVMM), or even a specific supplement for an individual micronutrient.

Do not forget that if you are getting sufficient amounts of these micronutrients from whole foods, there is no need to supplement. It is just as easy to be deficient as it is to get too much of a nutrient.

THE PROBIOTIC

The probiotic is a supplement that is relatively new to the market, but is quickly becoming popular. Learning the word and its roots helps you understand what it is designed to do. Basically, it is the opposite of the antibiotic, which kills bacteria. The probiotic promotes bacterial health in the gut, a key component in how the body absorbs ingested food. Once the food passes through the stomach it reaches the beginning of the intestinal tract. This is where the majority of absorption takes place, and it is not just a role of the intestinal cells that line the intestines, it is mostly facilitated by the gut biome, which is a culture of bacteria that live in the intestinal tract. The gut biome can also be referred to as the gut microbiota or the gut flora. They are the large community of bacteria that live in your lower Gastrointestinal (GI) tract, and one of the many roles they hold is in assisting nutrient yield from the foods you digest.

The main question is, why would it be beneficial to supplement this if the gut biome live there and already do their job? Before answering this we must consider just how important these bacterium are. To give a little perspective, they are actually considered a separate organ as they work together, have layers, subcomponents, and operate with common goals and functions as organs do with their composition of different tissues and cell types. These bacterium work beyond assisting in nutrient yield and absorption.

The main function outside of nutrient absorption is in immunity and assisting the host (you) with immune function. They essentially act as an additional layer of protection between the body's internal environment and what is basically toxic waste floating through the lower GI tract. That layer of gut bacterium works in conjunction with the gut immune tissues as a gatekeeper, and can be considered a key to maintaining the health of the entire body [43 – 45]. To bring a little light to the weight the gut carries in biological function, consider that the gut biome have ten times the rest of the body's DNA [46]. Knowing the sheer numbers of these organisms and the roles they play, we can begin to understand their importance.

The gut biome impact our functioning, and our nutrient intake impacts them. Note that the typical western diet does not positively impact the biome. A few examples are intakes of sugar, fat, and drugs. These things do not act alone on the flora, in fact, many times it is the culmination of food types and drugs that are most influential.

We also have to understand that the flora is something that has been a part of our biological functioning since early life, and is impacted by the birth delivery type, the infant's diet, hygiene, and administered medications during infantile life [47]. These impacts extend into adult life, but the early stage of human development is hugely impactful. As we grow, our medications, diet, and hygiene continue to influence the flora.

Have you ever taken an antibiotic? Chances are you have, but do you know how those impact the flora? There are many types of antibiotics, and they are prescribed for specific reasons, but all are generally prescribed to fight a bacterial infection. The problem with this is they not only fight the infection, but they also affect the good bacteria of the gut [48]. The type of antibiotic determines the interaction it has on the flora, but generally they change the flora's composition. With the important role played by the gut flora, we can see how this change may not be a good thing. It is not to say that antibiotics are bad, but they should be used properly and only when necessary to ensure the gut flora is not subjected to them unless it is required and done in the correct manner. Research indicates that antibiotics impact the gut microbe in a way that compromises the flora and facilitates intestinal infections [48].

All of this shows there could be a benefit to supplementing with something that promotes gut health. When you ingest a probiotic supplement you are essentially ingesting bacteria, the opposition of the antibiotic. Probiotic supplementation has been shown to positively impact the effects seen from a diet high in sugar, blunting the amplitudes of increases normally seen in blood sugar and fats [49]. These findings show how supplementation with a probiotic could possibly be beneficial to those that suffer from metabolic conditions, and how significant the gut biome is to general health. Other findings include improving immunity through improving the intestinal balance of the flora. Manifesting in improvements in food allergies, inflammatory conditions, and the improvement of the function of the gut's immune barrier [50]. Due to the function of the biome and considering how impactful absorption and immunity are across the entire host, there are many downstream benefits that can be postulated. In fact, there has even been a recent study that investigated a specific probiotic on male sexual health which showed improved hormonal levels and increased fertility during use of the probiotic [51].

There are different forms of the biotic supplements -- probiotic, prebiotic, and symbiotic and different strains of the bacterium. The importance of the gut biome cannot be discounted, but when considering a supplement, it is not advisable to go out and grab just any product off the shelf. There are many bacterium that make up the gut flora, and increasing one will impact others. The different forms also have different levels of effectiveness, and this should be taken into account. It is very important that these considerations be a part of the decision process of choosing whether to use a pro-, pre-, or symbiotic supplement. They may have implications for application, but there are a multitude of variables [52]. The more appropriate way to improve or "supplement" gut function is feeding it fiber from carbohydrate foods. In fact, dietary fiber is often used as an ingredient in biotic supplements. This is because dietary fiber is fermented and feeds the biome [53]. Supplementation can be an option but feeding the biome what it needs via carbohydrate and its fiber content should be viewed as the gold standard.

FISH OIL

Another common supplement is fish oil, or omega fatty acids. These are actually unsaturated essential fatty acids. These fatty acids are called essential because the body cannot make them and we need them from an outside source, just like the essential amino acids. They are found in the largest concentrations within fatty fish like salmon and tuna, among others. Fish oil pills are the same color as dietary oils. That is because it is an oil, or a less-than-solid fat, at room temperature. In fact, if you were to break one of these capsules the contents would spill out and would appear like the fat you would see in fish.

In *Healthy Body, Healthy Mind, Healthy Life Part I: Nutrition* we discovered that dietary fats may be more important than they once were thought to be. That includes the types of fats found in fish oil supplements. In fact, recent studies have explored the benefits associated with including a fish oil supplement in dietary intake. They have found that with supplementation the body is able to adapt to exercise stimuli to a greater degree.

One of the many impacts that chronic exercise has is on bone mineral density (BMD). Most research on fish oil supplementation is done in animals; one specific investigation looked into fish oil's impact on bone mass, density, formation, and resorption in aged rats with removed ovaries. The investigation showed that the supplementation had positive impacts on bone [54]. This provides implications for potential benefit to post-menopausal women considering the biological parameters. This has significant implications, since BMD is on a natural decline as a result of the aging process. These findings are even more significant for females considering estrogen dynamics following menopause. This investigation simply says that there is potential in the use of fish oil supplementation on bone health.

On top of that, there is increased ability in protein synthesis, improved immune function, and improved vascular health.

Research indicates that through a specific change in a signaling mechanism, fish oil supplementation allows the body to maintain and build more muscle [55]. It may also improve the immune response [56] and the health of the body's vessels. What was most significant in the study that investigated vascular impacts was that the use of fish oil decreased the risk of stroke. It did this by decreasing plaque accumulation and decreasing inflammation in the vessels of the brain, in a rat model [57]. It can be said that fish oil supplementation generally provides an anti-inflammatory impact.

Because of the benefits provided by this supplement, its use can be beneficial for a range of individuals. It has implications for increasing the body's response to exercise in ways that could improve performance and body composition, and also has implications for improving health status. With the effect on immunity, BMD, protein synthesis, and vessel health, this supplement could benefit the aging population where these things are on a natural decline as a result of the aging process. The benefits may also be applicable to people of all ages.

PROTEIN SUPPLEMENTS

The association of protein intake and exercise is well founded on the many functions dietary protein plays in the body. It is easy to see value in increasing protein intake, even from supplemental forms. In the previous chapter we discussed some of the dynamics of dietary protein and identified that the current research supports the range of 1.4 – 2.0 grams per kilogram of bodyweight per day in active, exercising adults. What has not been discussed are the different forms of supplemental protein available. Let's look at the different forms and the considerations that should be made when choosing a protein supplement.

There are many sources of supplemental protein. Some of the available sources on the market include whey, casein, egg, soy, pea, and rice. These sources are used as the major component of many protein supplements. Keep in mind all proteins are combinations of amino acids. The reason the listed types are used as protein products is because in their whole food forms they provide good sources of those amino acids.

The plant sources of supplemental protein can be a good way to increase total protein intake and enhance an exercise regimen. In fact, in one study researchers found that there was not a significant difference in the response seen between supplemental forms of whey and rice proteins in an eight week resistance training protocol [58]. This has implications for vegetarian and other restricted dietary programs in completing protein requirements, but we must still note that these proteins are highly processed. Knowing that information about rice is important when we look at the most popular supplemental plant-based protein, soy.

Since soy is one of the few complete plant proteins (in whole food form) and rice is incomplete, it would be logical to think that supplemental soy has a greater impact than rice, but in fact the opposite is true. In comparison to supplementing with casein (a complete milk protein), soy protein has been found to have a much less significant impact on the primary muscle synthetic pathway. However, it should be noted that most supplemental versions of soy are actually incomplete. Processed soy products are missing and low in the essential amino acids methionine and lysine, respectively. Soy products are also low in other non-essential amino acids.

It seems this low quality amino acid availability manifests in less protein synthesis, when soy is compared to other supplemental proteins [23]. This is not to discount soy protein, because it does have many potential benefits, including lowering LDL cholesterol, reducing the risk of various cardiovascular complications, and reduction of menopausal symptoms. These benefits may be due to the presence of the phytoestrogens (isoflavones) and their action on estrogen receptors [59]. However, it should be noted that there are mixed findings when studying soy and isoflavones in relation to breast cancer; some reports indicate reduction in risk while others report negative effects [60]. Though it should be noted that more recent analysis of epidemiology data on soy intake indicates no correlation between breast cancer in women in Western countries, however soy isoflavone intake may lower risk of breast cancer for both pre- and post-menopausal women in Asian countries [61]. Additionally, the myth that soy protein will negatively affect testosterone or other associated hormones in men is false [62]

The two most common types of supplemental protein sources are whey and casein, both of which are found naturally in milk. They are complete proteins and have great availability of amino acids [59]. Leucine is a key amino acid and whey and casein are good sources of it. They both stimulate protein synthesis and provide a great nutritional method of enhancing adaptation to exercise.

If they are both a good way to do this, why do some people say one is better than the other, and are there differences that need to be considered when selecting one? The most simple answer to that question is yes, there are differences and things to be considered when choosing between whey or casein. Whey acts faster and casein acts slower. They are both digested in about the same amount of time, however, due to the way casein clumps it is slower in releasing amino acids to the muscles once it is in the blood. With this slow release, casein is able to elevate the amino acids in the blood for longer than whey [63]. The slow release by casein provides the muscle with a constant supply of amino acids that can last for hours. This is a quality of casein that can be taken advantage of. The best way to do that would be to use it when there will be an extensive amount of time before the next meal, like before going to bed or if you are spacing out meals. Because of this characteristic there is a difference in the immediate stimulation of protein synthesis between casein and whey, where whey causes a greater immediate effect.

This is why it is considered optimal to use whey for the post-exercise protein intake.

Whey is typically the protein used in post exercise-related protein supplementation. One reason for that is its great leucine content and because of that is an amazing way to stimulate protein synthesis. But the body does require all the essential amino acids for optimal protein synthesis. Because whey is a great source for all essential amino acids, has good leucine content, and those amino acids are available to the muscle faster than they would be from casein, it is the better option when immediate exercise recovery is the purpose of the supplement.

The rate of release of the amino acids is a very important consideration when evaluating whey. If you recall, current research has debunked the idea of the anabolic window. As long as the leucine threshold is met within six hours of the cessation of the exercise, then optimum protein synthesis can take place. As a consideration, we look at how fast whey dumps its amino acids into the blood. This is done at such a fast rate that not all of them are used in protein synthesis, instead a portion may be used for energy [64]. There are pools of amino acids in the blood and cells. If those locations are full and there is no place for them to go, they will be turned into new sugar or used for energy production. This may sound like a bad thing, but it is not. The muscle can directly metabolize specific amino acids, and it requires energy to perform protein synthesis and build new muscle.

When using supplemental whey, it may be the case that there is not efficiency in utilizing the amino acids, but this is dependent on other variables in the diet. It does not negate the fact that the use of whey protein with resistance and other modes of exercise reduces the damaging effects of exercise and can improve muscle recovery. These things need to be considered, especially if the goals are specific enough. In fact, the differences in the release of the amino acids following ingestion of whey or casein are directly related to the magnitude of immediate protein synthesis; where whey has been found to increase blood levels of that key amino acid leucine more than casein does [65].

With whey holding the weight it does in the nutrition, supplementation, and performance realm, it has been highly studied and there have been many attempts to improve its use. This has manifested in some alternate forms. They include whey isolate, whey concentrate, and hydrolyzed whey.

If we look at the different names of the whey manipulations and break down the words used to classify them we can better asses what they might be. Doing this we now have isolated whey, concentrated whey, and hydrolyzed whey, which helps us understand what may have been done to change the original protein. One was isolated, one was concentrated, and one was hydrolyzed.

First, concentrated whey is simply the processing of the protein to provide a more concentrated dose per serving, with the end goal of creating a greater protein synthetic response. The processing removes some nutrients form the original milk protein to allow this greater concentration and provide a more biologically active protein source [64]. The most important thing that is removed is some of the lactose, or milk sugar. This may be beneficial for those looking to reduce the sugar content of their whey, but it may not be significant enough of a removal to provide a benefit to those that are lactose intolerant. These things can make whey concentrate an attractive product.

Isolated whey is a theoretical step above the concentrated product. It provides an even more concentrated amount of whey protein per serving because the processing takes out more of the other nutrients. Unlike the concentrate, the isolate has a significant enough of the lactose removed to be of benefit to the lactose intolerant individual [64]. Whey Isolates are considered the purest whey protein sources available because of the removal of the lactose, fat, and other constituents. They can contain 90% or greater concentrations of protein. The issue is that processing is done to such a degree that it causes damage to the proteins and may make them less effective for biological use. Whey concentrate has less protein but more of it is biologically available, while whey isolate has greater concentrations that are not as available for use, and isolates contains negligible lactose [64].

The hydrolyzed whey is yet another theoretical step up on the other types. We can see the prefix hydro- and therefore gather that it has something to do with water. We can also see the suffix is lyse, or lyze, which means to cut or cleave. Essentially, the protein molecules are cut into shorter chains of amino acids. The idea behind this whey protein is that the body has to do less work to absorb the amino acids that are ingested. It is a great idea, but with the debunking of the anabolic window, making the release of amino acids faster than whey is already capable of really provides no benefit. In general, the hydrolyzed whey is not necessarily superior to the other types. You also have to consider that this protein is even further processed than the isolate. With that we can hypothesize that the hydrolyzed is damaged even more, making it less bioavailable than the isolate.

Understanding the differences between these proteins is important, but it may be just as important to understand that whey and casein come from the same whole food, milk. If you prefer to stay with whole foods and are not lactose intolerant, milk is good source for both the fast whey and slow casein. There are many considerations to be made when choosing protein sources, and one of them may be convenience. If that is a big one, then the powdered or prepackaged supplemental forms can be a good way to ensure you are meeting your daily needs. But, supplemental protein should only be viewed as a way of meeting your daily protein needs (1.4 – 2.0g per kilogram of body weight per day).

BCAAs (Branched Chain Amino Acids)

Branched Chain Amino Acid (BCAA) supplements are a common supplement associated with exercise. They can be seen in many formulations, from free standing to other types.

Notice that the term amino acid is actually in the name. This is because these three amino acids are the only ones that have a branched structure and the only ones that the muscle cells can directly metabolize to produce that energy molecule, ATP. The BCAAs are leucine, iso-leucine, and valine. It is important to recognize that leucine's role in protein synthesis signaling.

Knowing that amino acids are the building blocks of protein structures and that the BCAAs have specific functions in the muscle cell, it is easy to see how they can have an association to muscle repair and growth. When you ingest a whole protein from any food it can have up to four levels of structure, although this depends on the type of protein and food ingested. With four levels you can imagine breaking the protein down into its individual building blocks is not an immediate occurrence. In fact, this breakdown is not complete until the food has reached the small intestines. Depending on the source, that can take as long as six hours. That said, providing your body the individual amino acid instead of the full four-structured protein allows for fast absorption, and therefore facilitates quick delivery to the amino acid pools. However, you should know you get this quick delivery from protein supplements as well.

This partly why BCAA supplements has become popular. They are seen in pre-workout, intra-work out, and post-workout formulas, as well as other supplements. They provide that immediate source of amino acids the muscle can use for energy production or aid in countering muscle protein breakdown. To amplify the understanding of the balancing act between protein synthesis breakdown, we consider the amino acid pools. Keeping these pools full for the cells to perform life-sustaining protein synthesis and exercise-associated protein synthesis is essential. If they run low then the body has to find somewhere else to take them from. The body uses basic logic, and asks the following question "What tissue do I not need to survive?" The answer is skeletal muscle, it is constantly burning up the body's precious energy and so when amino acids run low in the body, it will take amino acids out of it. If building lean mass is a goal, allowing that to happen will only make that goal harder to reach.

Looking at the BCAA and its key component, leucine, we must ask why this is better than drinking a protein supplement or eating a whole food that provides the adequate amount of BCAAs. Research supports that the body only requires 1.8 to 3.5 grams of leucine to maximally stimulate protein synthesis [66, 67], however you should know that all things in the body are relative. In this case it means that the larger you are the more leucine you will need to meet this threshold. Considering the leucine threshold, calories in and calories out becomes a part of the equation. If you have a fat loss goal, then the BCAA supplement can be a way to go as they are typically low in calories but may aid in minimizing protein breakdown.

Another thing to consider about the leucine threshold is research indicates that meeting it before a workout actually provides a greater magnitude of protein synthesis than meeting it after [68]. This does provide support for the use of a stand-alone BCAA supplement before a workout to influence protein breakdown and synthesis.

Many BCAA containing supplements will have certain amounts of leucine, iso-leucine, and valine in them but it is really only leucine you need to pay attention to. At times you will see amounts that do not cause the optimal biological response. Recall, the leucine threshold is 1.8 to 3.5 grams per serving. In cases where the leucine content is less than that, one would have to take more than one serving to see the purported benefits. I have heard of people adding BCAAs to a protein source or taking BCAAs with a meal. This is improper, most meals containing protein foods and protein supplements will already provide the amount of BCAAs without adding extra. The only meal type I can think of that could benefit from the addition of BCAA ingestion is vegetarian, and even plant-based meals contain varying foods that complement each other's amino acid content.

Branched Chain Amino Acid supplements are often used to aid in the fasting window. While the logic is valid, intaking amino acids causes an insulin response and completely negates the health effects that many are trying to receive from a fast. Not to mention the protein synthetic response one gets from BCAAs is, at most, protective against protein breakdown.

Leucine is important, research suggests that in the presence of the same amount of leucine across different types of protein sources, the magnitude of protein synthesis is similar [58]. Even in the presence of low protein and adequate leucine, protein synthesis can be optimized [69]. However, it should be noted that in this and the previously cited investigation all essential amino acids are present, and all EAAs are needed to maximally stimulate the muscle synthetic response [23, 67, 70, 71]. This research basically indicates that if you want to supplement with amino acids the product needs to contain all nine essential amino acids to optimize protein synthesis.

It really comes down to goals, convenience, calories, and what you can afford. For most people the BCAA supplement is a waste of money.

CREATINE

Creatine is a biological compound that is very well known in supplementation. To understand how creatine is used we must go to the basics of energy in the body. The ATP molecule is composed of one adenosine and three phosphates bonded together. In muscle contraction, the separation of that third phosphate and the breaking of the chemical bond releases energy. We can posit that how the body stores and replenishes ATP is a very significant factor in the continuation of muscle contraction. This becomes especially significant in those stronger, non-fatigue resistant fibers that are classified as the Type-II x.

A little background on the fiber types will help us understand why this is the case. Skeletal muscle fibers have been put into three classifications for comparison and research purposes: Type-I, Type-IIa, and Type-IIx. The Type-I are also known as slow twitch fibers, while the Type-IIa and x are both considered fast twitch fibers. This means the Type-I are very resistant to fatigue and can continually contract in aerobic production of ATP. The Type-II are just the opposite, they can only contract for a short period of time before they begin to fatigue and exhaust their ATP, and they generally rely more on anaerobic replenishment of this ATP. The Type-II fibers are separated into a and x because they are similar but not exactly the same. Type-IIa can continue contraction for longer than IIx, but less powerfully however are slightly more aerobic than the IIx. Basically, IIa is the inbetween fiber of Type-I and IIx.

The range of fatigue resistance that is seen between the fiber types is based on microanatomy and the composition of the fibers; essentially they are classified by their metabolic and neural characteristics. They all have the same basic anatomy, but the amount of, lack of, or presence of different structures or even different versions of structures determines how the fiber produces energy and uses fuel. On a generalized level, the Type-I fibers use more fats to produce ATP, the Type-IIa use more carbohydrates to produce ATP, and the Type-IIx use stored ATP and creatine phosphate.

With this very general breakdown of the differences in fuel production, use, and composition of the muscle fiber types, we can look more at the role of creatine and creatine phosphate. The Type-IIx fibers are known for their explosive and powerful contractions. Exercises that require use of these fibers are those that that last a maximum of around 15 seconds, such as Olympic lifting or maximal sprinting. After the Type-IIx can no longer perform all out explosive contraction, the Type-IIa become more dominant. This is because a whole muscle is comprised of all types of fibers, just in different amounts. They contract to assist each other and keep the body moving.

The Type-IIx performs its contraction by using its stores of ATP within the muscle, which only accounts for that initial 2-4 seconds of activity. The difference in the 2-4 and 15 seconds is made by creatine and the PCr system. Creatine is used in this PCr system, or the Phosphocreatine system. Creatine is stored and attached to a phosphate within the cell so it may be used. This molecule is used to transport the phosphate to the ADP (one adenosine and two phosphates) and make it an ATP so that the muscle fiber can continue to contract in a powerful manner beyond that 2-4 seconds.

We can only get a limited amount of creatine from the diet, and if you are not eating the right kinds of foods chances are your intramuscular creatine is not anywhere near its full capacity. Foods that contain the most creatine are meat sources. There are some plants that contain it, but it is minimal compared to meats. Animals are better sources of the three amino acids arginine, glycine, and methionine, which are used to synthesize creatine [72]. This is why the vegetarian and other plant-based diets are lacking on creatine ingestion.

If the diet is not high enough in these foods, then the body will not be able to efficiently saturate the muscle with creatine. This alone provides implications for how creatine supplementation can impact performance in someone that utilizes a plant-based diet, but even in a meat eater creatine supplementation can be beneficial. This is because the body is constantly excreting creatine in its waste. In fact, the numbers are as follows: the average dietary intake of an omnivore is one to two grams per day, there are then small amounts synthesized by the liver and kidneys (depending on the diet zero to two grams), and then two to four grams are excreted daily [73, 74].

We can see how it may be difficult to maintain adequate amounts of intramuscular creatine, but since ninety-five percent is maintained in the muscle, it is important for that exercising population. Creatine supplementation has also safely been used in people with a number of health complications [75]; it plays a significant role in cellular energy.

Increasing the body's amount of creatine increases the capacity of the PCr system. This is the reason creatine can be used in exercise to improve performance. It is the most highly studied type of supplementation. These studies have again and again suggested that it does improve short, powerful exercise performance [75]. This is why it is one of the most highly used supplements on the market and is commonly added into other supplements like pre-workout formulations.

While there are great benefits to creatine, there have also been some claims of risks involved in consuming it; however these are mostly myths. Let's first outline the common myths and misconceptions of creatine supplementation. The most common myths are the following: all weight gained during supplementation is due to water retention; creatine supplementation causes renal (kidney) distress; it causes cramping, dehydration, and/or altered electrolyte status; long-term effects of creatine supplementation are completely unknown; newer creatine formulations are more beneficial than creatine monohydrate and cause fewer side effects; creatine supplementation is unethical and/or illegal. Reviews of the research on creatine supplementation show that these are all misconceptions [76].

The evidence does not support that creatine is damaging or provides negative side effects in healthy people. In fact, the research on creatine supplementation has shown benefits to the following populations: neurodegenerative diseases, diabetes, osteoarthritis, fibromyalgia, aging, brain and heart ischemia, adolescent depression, and pregnancy [75]. The misconceptions surrounding creatine are just those, misconceptions. That being the case, what else is there to know about creatine?

First and foremost, the original supplemental form is Creatine Monohydrate (CM). There have been other forms produced to try to increase the effectiveness and decrease some of those claimed negative consequences, including Creatine Ethyl Ester (CEE), Creatine Hydrochloric Acid (HCl), Micronized Creatine (MCC), and Kre-Alkalyn Creatine. The current data have studied primarily CM and there is not sufficient data to suggest other forms outperform CM in any parameter [76].

There is potentially some benefit to the other forms in regards to gastric distress, because some individuals do experience this when ingesting CM on an empty stomach. However, this can be avided by not consuming creatine on an empty stomach. The common belief that creatine has to be ingested before or right after exercise (when the stomach is empty) is not true. Creatine does not provide acute exercise benefits, and benefits are only seen with chronic ingestion [77]. The purpose of CM supplementation is to increase whole body concentrations by saturating the skeletal muscle. It can be taken at any time during and should be taken with meals, preferably meals that contain carbohydrate. Doing this may even help with any issues digesting CM.

Secondly, the same misconception that is associated with high protein intake is associated with CM supplementation, it is bad for the kidneys. As we learned previously, high protein intake is not associated with comprised kidney health in those that have healthy kidneys. This holds true with CM supplementation. In a review of studies that covered investigations of supplementing for five days, nine weeks, and as long as five years, there were no adverse effects on kidney function with any of these lengths of CM supplementation [78].

The next idea surrounding CM is that it dehydrates, changes electrolyte balance, or causes water retention. Yes, there can be weight gain via muscle mass during CM supplementation, but it is often thought to be due to the idea of bloating or water retention. The fact is these things are not true. Creatine is a molecule that attracts water, so as the intramuscular concentration goes up there is a change in the water distribution between the body's water compartments, both intracellular and extracellular. This means that as more creatine gets stored in the muscle cell so does more water [79, 80], leaving less in the extracellular area.

It does not cause dehydration, change electrolyte balance, or cause weight gain via water retention. In fact, the weight gain that is seen is caused by the increased ability to perform high-intensity work by the muscle. The muscle's ability to perform greater work allows for greater adaptation as a result of the increased work output [76]. Although, because there is less water in the extracellular area it may be beneficial to increase water intake to offset the change in water distribution.

Understanding the misconceptions and knowing that CM is a way to increase high-intensity exercise performance, let's look more at application. All fiber types use the PCr system for ATP replenishment. We only gave the explosive Type-IIx example because that fiber type uses it to the highest degree. Other fibers use it as an intermediate of energy production as intensities are changing, so the cell can replenish ATP while it is waiting for the other energy faucets to "kick in". One example would be a marathon runner's muscles using creatine and the PCr when she has to go from running on a flat surface to running up a hill (or even standing up from your chair). Putting more creatine in the muscle allows greater intensities to be performed for longer periods of time in all types of exercise. In short, creatinine can be used to increase exercise performance without causing any adverse effects in healthy people [75].

As far as dosing goes the broad base recommendation is consuming 3-5 grams per day. There is a protocol for loading but in my opinion that is a waste of the supplement. Adaptation takes time so commit to the training. If you decided to include creatine in your regimen take it daily with meals and that will be enough to increase your muscular stores.

PRE-WORKOUT SUPPLEMENTS

One of the most commonly used supplements is the pre-workout supplement. The marketing says it will give you that extra pump or rush of energy to get you started. These are probably some of the most common supplements next to protein.

Some common ingredients found in pre-workout formulas are: creatine, beta-alanine, L-arginine, thiamin (vitamin B1), riboflavin (vitamin B2), niacin (vitamin B3), and caffeine.

First creatine, a supplement that works effectively to increase the muscle fiber's potential to create a greater amount of work and perform that level of work for a longer period of time than it would have without the outside source of creatine. Recall the PCr system and ATP replenishment. Just as the body uses the macronutrients in the energy faucets, the different fibers use ATP stores, the PCr system, anaerobic, and aerobic ATP production similarly. This is because these and the energy faucets are related.

The fibers all have the ability to use these pathways and sources of ATP. The specific pathway and its use is dependent on what type of fiber, what activity it is performing, and the intensity and duration of that activity. This makes creatine seem like a great additive to a pre-workout formula, but recall that timing of creatine ingestion is not significant, it is the chronic saturation of the skeletal muscle that matters [77]. That said, it is not needed in a pre-workout formula. It is needed in daily consumption.

The next two items listed are beta-alanine (Beta or β) and L-arginine. These are actually amino acids. These two are reportedly associated with enhancement of muscular function during exercising conditions. β -alanine is associated with acid-base balance in buffering acidic byproducts created during exercise [81], while L-arginine is associated with vessel dilation and increased blood flow [82].

Because of the physiological functioning, beta is a very common supplement either in pre-workout formulas or free standing. When beta is introduced to the body it is digested and eventually is circulated in the blood. There the muscles are able to take it in and combine it with L-histidine, an additional amino acid, to make carnosine. Carnosine is the major intracellular hydrogen buffer. Hydrogen is a major byproduct of exercise metabolism and its accumulation causes a negative change in muscle pH, this is the burn you feel. Carnosine is able to buffer the internal pH of the muscle to allow greater work to be done by the muscle before the pH inhibits its action [81].

Beta is an effective component of pre-workout formulas because it allows the muscle to work harder for longer periods in high-intensity conditions. The research supports that the best results are seen in high-intensity bouts that last one to four minutes due to the action it has on positively impacting exercise-related pH in the muscle. It is like creatine in that it takes daily consumption to see the benefits. In order to see those benefits one must consume four to six grams per day for at least two to four weeks [81]. If you are taking a pre-workout supplement that has the right amounts (most don't), but you don't take it every day because you don't train every day, chances are you are not seeing the full benefit of beta supplementation.

L-arginine is associated with the urea cycle and increasing production of nitric oxide (NO) [82, 83]. Nitric oxide falls into the classification of a vessel dilator or vasodilator. Vasodilators increase blood flow by increasing the diameter of vessels, thereby decreasing the pressure the walls of the vessels apply to blood flow. Originally it was thought that L-arginine would aid in how fast by-products of exercise metabolism are moved out of local muscular areas and allow the heart to pump a greater amount of blood to a muscle that needs it. The problem with L-arginine is that the research does not support these benefits because it is broken down in the stomach before it can perform its purported claims.

There is current research supporting the use L-citrulline because it is not broken down before it gets into the blood. It can make it into the urea cycle and cause increases in blood NO [84]. L-arginine does not provide the benefits it was originally thought to, while L-citrulline does [85]. Using a pre-workout supplement that contains citrulline can be of benefit, but this ingredient is like others in that it requires the appropriate dose. Though there is not a specific dose that is agreed upon by the scientist, the studies that have been done using citrulline use dosages between 4 and 6 grams [86]. If you see dose that is below that you may want to choose another product. Additionally, if the product lists citrulline malate the dosage has to be divided by two, so 6g of citrulline malate is 3g of citrulline and 3g of malate.

The next set of common ingredients are the major B vitamins: thiamin (vitamin B1), riboflavin (vitamin B2), and niacin (vitamin B3). These are the big three B vitamins and co-enzymes in macronutrient metabolism. Their role in energy and bioenergetics is why they are included in pre-workout formulas. As you can imagine, energy metabolism goes up incredibly during exercise. The role of these become crucial as they increase a cell's macronutrient energy harvesting of carbohydrates, fats, and proteins.

If you have ever taken a pre-workout supplement you have probably heard about or experienced the rush or flush of the skin. If the supplement contains Beta above 1.6 grams per serving it has the potential to cause that tingling feeling, paresthesia, however it has no harmful impacts [81]. This flushing feeling can also come from a toxic dose of water-soluble B vitamins. B1 can have what is called a cholinergic effect [87]. This is where the vitamin allows the body to produce a major biological component, acetylcholine. It seems that the tingling feeling from a pre-workout provides no actual benefit other than psychological, however, if the tingling is from B vitamins it could be a sign of a toxic dose.

B2 and B3 are used by the body to synthesize electron transporters. These are used in metabolism in the final steps of synthesizing ATP aerobically. B1, 2, and 3 are needed for optimal metabolic activity, but research has not found a benefit of supplementing them when getting enough from a balanced diet [88]. However, this is a very understudied area of sport nutrition.

The final major ingredient is caffeine. Caffeine is widely known for its role as an energy booster and is often associated with fat burning. In fact, it is highly studied in this realm.

To understand why caffeine is as highly regarded as it is in sports supplementation we must first look at how it works, starting with consumption. Once it reaches the GI tract it is absorbed and chemically digested, resulting in three metabolites that circulate the blood and cause its effects. These do not peak in the blood until about one hour after ingestion. At that point they can act on the body's tissues and are not cleared out for about three to six hours. The action of the metabolites is not completely understood, however they are able to pass through the membrane of cells, so their impact on the body is great. The two tissues that are studied the most are neural and muscular [89].

The most significant action these metabolites have are on adenosine receptors in the brain. If you recall the ATP energy molecule, the A represents the adenosine backbone, which shows how caffeine has a relationship to biological energy dynamics. Caffeine blocks adenosine from binding to these receptors. When adenosine attaches to its receptor it results in reactions that promote sleepiness. In that, caffeine positively impacts energy perception.

Caffeine is able to act on these by permeating the blood brain barrier (BBB). Additionally, caffeine's metabolites pass through all membranes and act on all tissues [90]. Acting on the muscle and Central Nervous System (CNS) is hugely impactful on exercise.

Due to the ability to act on the CNS and nervous tissue, caffeine is very influential, from energy to cognition. It is able to increase fat metabolism and decrease carbohydrate metabolism, in resting conditions [91]. It is able to increase the release of endorphins from the brain [92]. In exercise, that allows the individual to work harder because of lower perceived amounts of exercise induced discomfort [93]. It even impacts muscular contraction dynamics, and seems to allow the muscle to reach its maximum contractile force with a less significant stimulus [94].

These are all important things to know but also sound like common sense if you have ever used a pre-workout supplement or even coffee. What needs to be addressed is how to evaluate the dose in a supplement. The literature suggests the best dosage is 3-6mg per kilogram of bodyweight [89]. To find what that means for you divide your weight by 2.2 and then multiply by 3 and 6. This will give you the range in milligrams that is optimal for your performance. You can use that to evaluate a supplement's dose. It is also important to know that caffeine, caffeine containing compounds, and caffeine isomers (versions of caffeine) can be seen on the same label as anhydrous caffeine, natural caffeine, tea extracts, guarana, guayusa, di-caffeine malate, caffeine citrate, dynamine, and others.

Of course, there are many other things that could be discussed but knowing what to look for on a label is a good starting point.

ANABOLIC AGENTS

Anabolic agents are more commonly called steroids, so we need a little clarification before diving into this topic. Within the body steroids include an entire class of hormones, and these hormones are cholesterol based. For example estradiol, which is the main estrogen, and cortisol, a catabolic hormone, are both steroid hormones. Therefore we need to distinguish between those that elicit the physiological changes of which we are talking about. These are compounds that are primarily testosterone derived and are related to signaling anabolic pathways, for the purposes of this we will refer to them as anabolics.

Anabolics are all designed around the goal of increasing size, strength, or performance in some capacity related to increasing protein synthesis and structure building, and therefore muscle performance. This is the impact of the primary male androgen, testosterone. It is anabolic and is associated with the development of the primary male characteristics. That being the case, the most popular use of anabolic agents seems to be sources and derivatives of testosterone [95].

Knowing these things, we can gather how anabolics could possibly result in increased sports performance and body composition adaptations. These anabolics are not to be confused with compounds or herbs that claim to improve free testosterone. These free testosterone boosters are those that claim to stimulate the body to make more of its own free testosterone. For example, the herb tribulus theoretically does this. This concept of the anabolic is surrounded by a huge dark cloud of negative attention.

First, you have probably read or heard something that says anabolics are bad. There are often many questions concerning anabolic use. What is it that the research actually finds to be true, and what are the variables of these studies? How many studies have been performed on anabolics in comparison to legal drugs, like tobacco or alcohol? Did you know that when you are hospitalized for trauma you are given steroids to enhance your body's ability to heal damaged tissues? These questions are not asked to provide support to a pro-steroid argument, instead I want to get you thinking about the topic from an objective point of view. With that, what about the health perspective? How does the use of anabolics impact the health status of the numerous physiological systems? Why do the populations that are associated with use tend to die at a relatively young age? What are the reasons that the association of use is always negative?

It is largely understood that the use of anabolics is illegal in many sports and frowned upon in others, but there are industries that thrive on their use. This mainly seen in strength sport athletes and physique competitors. While there are competitions that are all-natural, implying that there is no use of anabolics, there are also many competitions that do not hold any standards on use. This is where the largest amount of anabolic use is thought to be found, but there are also regular gym goers and many others that use them.

Genetics, maturation, exercise programming, total caloric intake, macronutrient distributions, and recovery are key foundations for achieving the goals that surround the use of anabolics and muscle performance. Once these things are properly established, the use of an anabolic may have the potential to enhance goal attainment, but a good foundation in the other elements is required, first.

The functions of circulating testosterone on the tissues range. Anabolic signaling is one of the major functions, and it is joined by muscle metabolism, growth hormone stimulation, neurotransmitter dynamics, and impacts on the nervous system [96, 97]. Hormones and hormonal interactions are highly variable, and testosterone has the potential to be very influential on other hormones. Knowing that testosterone has a relationship with muscle growth, muscle metabolism, and the control system of the body (the nervous system), we can begin to understand that outside sources above normal blood concentrations have the potential to greatly influence exercise performance and body composition.

The application of levels that exceed normal physiological testosterone have been found to improve muscle size, strength, and body composition [98]. The degree to which these adaptations occur are variable from individual to individual, but even in the case where the use of testosterone is applied without a heavy resistance training program, there are changes in the body composition seen where there is an increase in lean mass. Even though this is the case, it is dependent on the dose of the anabolic.

One very significant thing that testosterone does is impact what are called satellite cells. Satellite cells are the stem cells of muscle. They are responsible for growth and development when we are developing new muscle tissue during our younger years. After that, they are only really stimulated to repair muscle damage. For our purposes, we are considering exercise induced damage.

The amplitude of satellite cell stimulation is affected by the contraction type. Eccentric contractions, which is the lengthening of a muscle, seem to cause more damage, and through that damage cause greater stimulation of satellite cells [99]. If you have ever done negatives and experienced the amount of soreness that follows, then you have experienced a manifestation of that damage. That muscle damage causes greater growth through the stimulation of satellite cells, even without the application of anabolics. Use of testosterone, has been found to increase the amount of satellite cells in a muscle through satellite cell proliferation, therefore creating a greater capacity for muscle growth [100].

An additional thing to consider is the biological agent myostatin. Anything with the suffix -statin is an inhibitor and anything with the prefix myo- is referencing muscle. Essentially myostatin regulates the growth of skeletal muscle through inhibition [101]. Testosterone has been found to negatively regulate or decrease myostatin expression [102], which allows for greater growth of skeletal muscle. Basically, it negates our natural muscle growth limiter.

There are more satellite cells to be stimulated to cause growth of muscle tissue and there is less myostatin to limit that growth. These show us why anabolic use can facilitate growth and seem like great things for the athletic population or those looking for improved performance or body composition, but they also have implications for other populations.

As muscle atrophy is a natural part of aging, it is seen in a large majority of aging persons and if severe enough it can lead to sarcopenia. There has even been research to investigate this, showing that using outside sources of testosterone opposed the loss of muscle through its action on satellite cells and the development of more of those muscle stem cells [103]. This is not the only population that this type of supplementation has potential positive implications for; there are many conditions like muscular dystrophy and others that could potentially benefit from exogenous testosterone.

There is one other thing that is commonly associated with testosterone, which is male sexual health. Research has found that men who have compromised sexual health find a benefit in testosterone treatment, but that same benefit is not found in men that are otherwise sexually healthy [104]. In fact, there may be negative impacts on the body, including prostate health via testosterone therapy, where the prostate grows or hypertrophies as a result of the anabolic stimulus of high levels of an anabolic agent [105], even though there is a transient perceived improvement.

The majority of the adaptations that have been covered on the use of testosterone derivatives are in relation skeletal muscle, but this is not the only area are affected by testosterone use. There is a common idea that anabolics reduce the good cholesterol, HDL, but some evidence says that this may not be the case unless the administered amount is extremely high. In fact, a review of the research shows that there may be a reduced risk for atherosclerosis, Type-II Diabetes, fat accumulation in the viscera, and coronary artery disease with testosterone replacement in therapeutic doses [106]. That said, therapeutic doses are not the same as those that many use for recreational and performance purposes.

When it comes to anabolics, what must be considered is that these findings are the result of controlled studies. It is common to hear of body builders passing away from cardiovascular complications. With these individuals there may not be the same administered dosages that those in the controlled studies are receiving. They may be taking much more, or even using a technique called stacking, where multiple anabolic agents and drugs are used at high levels [107]. This technique changes the variables and has the potential to cause physiological adaptations which could increase the risk for things such as cardiovascular disease, heart attack, stroke, metabolic illness, changes in psychological health and many other negative complications.

Knowing that a stacking technique is common, we look next at the term roid rage; another negative connotation that surrounds the use of anabolics. This generally occurs in relation to a change in aggression or a negative change in psychological health that is a result of use of an anabolic drug. The research on this effect suggests that even when administered in levels that greatly shadow normal physiological testosterone, there is not an increase in aggressive behavior [108]. What needs to be considered about the research on this topic is that these are findings of apparently psychologically healthy men, and the result of survey data (self-reported) collection. With the consideration of the stacking technique and other variables, anabolic use does have the potential to elicit angry behavior and changes in mood, but these things are all dependent on individual application and may be largely influenced by the individual's psychological health prior to use.

We have identified testosterone and estradiol as androgens. They are the sex hormones, and they have very specific functions that sometimes oppose each other. With that opposing function they are maintained at specific levels to counter each other in the way they are biologically designed. The use of anabolic agents raises testosterone levels, but also has the potential to raise estrogen (estradiol) levels. Administering of testosterone has been shown to increase the circulating levels of estradiol [109]. This has been found to be dose and fat dependent, so the more testosterone administered and the higher the body fat percentage, the more estradiol rises when using testosterone. This is partially due to conversion of the extra testosterone to that main estrogen by an enzyme called aromatase. This is one of the reasons multiple drugs are used. To reduce the side effects of other drugs, the aromatase conversion, as well as an attempt to protect normal physiological function.

Using an outside source of testosterone can possibly be of benefit to many populations, from clinical cases and the elderly to performance and body composition. That does not mean there aren't risks. In introducing this exogenous testosterone (or other drugs), you are influencing one of the major physiological systems, the endocrine system. It regulates many things and influences the entire body as hormones travel through the blood to act on their targets. With the many interactions that occur between hormones, changing the circulating amounts has the potential to impact many things. Testosterone being the chief male androgen, is directly related to male sexual health and a variety of other bodily functions. The impact of high exogenous levels varies. There are ways to do it that reduce the risk, but there are always risks.

The importance of this is to address the fact that there is a plethora of anabolic agents and drugs on the market. They are seen as Androstendiol, Hydroxytestosterone, Methylandrostendione, Calusterone, Dehydrochlormethyltestosterone, Fluoxymesterone, Methandrostenolone, Oxabolone, Stenbolone, Trenbolone, and many others, but most are derivatives of testosterone or progesterone. There are many people that exercise in many different levels of experience that consider anabolic use as an option. The problem is that the large majority do not know what they are putting their body through.

Essentially what these things do is increase the body's ability to heal and grow exponentially but there is always a cost. The research in this area is limited and controversial. There is a lot that is not known or even being looked at because of the negative associations that come with the steroid and studying a human.

Yes, there are negative side effects with anabolics, but it is very difficult to say exactly what those are, especially with the amount of drugs available and all of the individual factors like diet, genetics, and dosages. In general, the negative effects for men include alteration of blood lipids, increased blood pressure (via increased red blood cell count), gynecomastia (breast development), hypogonadism (testicular atrophy), hair growth or loss, and acne. For women side effects include deepening voice, enlarged clitoris, irregular menstrual cycle (or cessation), and structural body changes. It is difficult to say what the long-term effects of these anabolic agents may be, due to the many individual factors at play, but for now we can see there are a lot of negative outcomes.

Earlier there were some questions posed about anabolic agents and the negative connotation. The problem with this type of supplement is that the consumer becomes addicted to the results. What if you went from a bench press of 185lbs to 245lbs in the matter of 6 to 8 weeks (or less), and also gained 15 pounds of lean muscle while losing fat? Considering where you started, you may feel like a super human. Let's put this in the perspective of a runner. What if you went from running a 5K at an eight minute mile pace to running that same course in a five minute mile pace? In this example you would have shaved off nine minutes from your total time; you may feel like a super human.

That is where the addiction comes, and the negative connotation follows. Individuals coming off a cycle may feel like they lose their gains, so they go back on the drugs with a larger dose. This has the potential of becoming a vicious cycle where the consumer wants more each time. This cycle turns into overuse and results in the negative attention placed on anabolics. If you decide that this is an option, you must understand the risks you are taking and be prepared to do in-depth research on how to do it correctly so do it with the lowest risk possible.

Also, know that this is just the tip of the iceberg when it comes to drug use for body composition and human performance. There are a lot more drugs out there and a lot of risk is placed on health when using drugs, especially when using a stacking method.

Recall genetics, maturation, exercise programming, total caloric intake, macronutrient distributions, and recovery are key foundations for achieving the goals that surround the use of anabolics and performance. If one decides that this is something they want to put their body through they must first establish the foundation in these, then own the fact that they are going to the extreme to meet their goals. If you don't you are going about it without recognizing the choice you are making.

5 SUPPLEMENTATION: THE BIG PICTURE

Supplements are widely associated with the resistance training community, and therefore there is a stigma that follows the word supplementation. But in reality, supplements are much more dynamic than they seem. Supplements apply to all ages and populations. For example, a newborn is given a shot of vitamin K, and an elderly adult may be administered a wide variety of supplements like intrinsic factor, which is essential for the absorption of vitamin B12. They are a viable option for many people, including those who have serious dietary restrictions like celiac disease. While there are benefits, it does not mean supplements are a good source of nutrition to make up for poor dietary choices. Simply put what supplements do is in the name - supplement dietary intake.

In the previous chapter we identified some of the most common forms of supplementation, but they aren't the only ones available. There are supplemental forms of every vitamin and mineral we know of, and we only covered the MVMM. We have also covered some popular supplements that claim to promote performance. It is important to understand that while there is research conducted on supplements, this is research conducted in the laboratory setting. That means there are controls, designs, and specific analysis tools utilized to measure the results and their meaning. It is also important to understand that you don't live in a lab, so the results you see may not be exactly what the label says. This is especially the case if you do not apply the supplement exactly the way it was applied during the research. Not to mention the placebo effect is a reality.

There are a range of types of supplements, but according to the International Society of Sports Nutrition (ISSN) there are four general categories:(I) Apparently Effective, (II) Possibly Effective, (III) Too Early To Tell, and (IV) Apparently Ineffective. Supplements are put into these categories based upon the evidence from research performed on that specific supplement [110], and a large majority do not get classified apparently effective.

When it comes to regulation, the supplement market is not as strict as the pharmacological market, but it is still regulated. In 1994 the Dietary Supplement Health and Education Act (DSHEA) was signed into law to provide regulation on dietary supplements. With the competitive marketplace that is the supplement market, there is a battle for companies to have return customers. The FDA and Federal Trade Commission (FTC) do set guidelines for these companies. The companies that follow the guidelines typically are able to compete in the marketplace at a higher level because the guidelines are designed around providing a safe and quality product [110]. Just because supplements are not directly regulated by the FDA does not mean they are unsafe.

SUPPLEMENTATION: THE LABEL

When it comes to supplement labels one thing to look out for is the FDA's Good Manufacturing Practices (GMP) seal. Some people have the impression that supplements contain ingredients that aren't good for them or may even be harmful, but in order for a company to be profitable and last in the marketplace it must develop and maintain a customer base. It only makes sense that a company does not harm their customers, because that could lead to bad press and investigations or costly law suits. In fact, many companies use third-party independent testing to ensure their product is safe and will provide the intended result. This is their safety net to make sure they are doing what they need to ensure they can keep customers coming back [110].

All of this does not negate the fact that the companies that sell supplements are looking to turn a profit by selling a product for more than they purchased it for. The regulations placed on these companies are pretty loose, even though they are there. You must find a company you trust to provide a good product that has what the label says it does.

When choosing a supplement, you also need to make sure the formulation makes sense for the desired outcome. This is mostly concerning the pre-workout, but it can generally be applied to the entire spectrum of sport supplementation. There is research that provides results for supplements used in specific situations that either suggests it works, doesn't work, or needs further investigation. Recall the four categories of supplements. Just as an example of application a specific study looked at pre-workout supplementation and found that in both males and females there was no difference in force production between the placebo and the supplement [111]. So, in that application (force production) there was no benefit but there could be a benefit to some other measure. Because of the specific focus of the study and measure it appears that that supplement does not have any real benefits, but we cannot say for sure that it is completely useless.

It is up to the company to use the right ingredients in the right amounts to provide the best result, but you must consider that most supplements actually do not provide a measurable benefit. There are only a handful that provide some type of increase in performance via objective testing. The supplements that really work are usually classified a drug. The ones that are not classified drugs but provide some benefit, like beta-alanine, are the ones that you see most commonly on the label. The problem is that in the majority of cases they are not in the right dosages. When that happens, the label is used as a way sell the product rather than the ingredients or the evidence. For example, it is possible to formulate a pre-workout supplement for the cardiovascular mode of training, however, this is not a common supplement. In fact, to make the best supplements for specific use it is advisable to purchase free standing ingredients and formulate your own.

There are many questions concerning supplementation and how the body responds or doesn't. The science is new and we are always learning new things about it. If you are considering adding supplementation to your nutritional intake and want to be serious about it, you should consult someone who specializes in sport nutrition. The gold standard certification in sports nutrition is awarded by the International Society of Sports Nutrition (ISSN) and is seen as the CISSN. There are many professionals out there, but those that have earned the CISSN, or other specialized certifications, higher education in sports nutrition, or licensure as a Registered Dietitian (RD) should be regarded as the authorities. Also, it should be noted the RD has more nutritional knowledge, especially of the clinical nature.

REFERENCES

1) ZOBEL, E. H., ET AL. (2016). "GLOBAL CHANGES IN FOOD SUPPLY AND THE OBESITY EPIDEMIC." CURR OBES REP 5(4): 449-455.

2) ZHAO, Y., ET AL. (2017). "FAST FOOD CONSUMPTION AND ITS ASSOCIATIONS WITH OBESITY AND HYPERTENSION AMONG CHILDREN: RESULTS FROM THE BASELINE DATA OF THE CHILDHOOD OBESITY STUDY IN CHINA MEGA-CITIES." BMC PUBLIC HEALTH 17(1): 933

3) ZHANG, N., ET AL. (2017). "CURRENT LIFESTYLE FACTORS THAT INCREASE RISK OF T2DM IN CHINA." EUR J CLIN NUTR 71(7): 832-838.

4) PADILLA, P. AND P. MIRAMONTES (2006). "A THEORETICAL FRAMEWORK FOR DEFINING SOME CONCEPTS IN EVOLUTION." RIV BIOL 99(2): 273-285.

5) BLAIR, S. N., ET AL. (1989). "PHYSICAL FITNESS AND ALL-CAUSE MORTALITY. A PROSPECTIVE STUDY OF HEALTHY MEN AND WOMEN." JAMA 262(17): 2395-2401.

6) LECKER, S. H., ET AL. (1999). "MUSCLE PROTEIN BREAKDOWN AND THE CRITICAL ROLE OF THE UBIQUITIN-PROTEASOME PATHWAY IN NORMAL AND DISEASE STATES." J NUTR 129(1S SUPPL): 227S-237S.

7) BORENSZTAJN, J. AND D. S. ROBINSON (1970). "THE EFFECT OF FASTING ON THE UTILIZATION OF CHYLOMICRON TRIGLYCERIDE FATTY ACIDS IN RELATION TO CLEARING FACTOR LIPASE (LIPOPROTEIN LIPASE) RELEASABLE BY HEPARIN IN THE PERFUSED RAT HEART." J LIPID RES 11(2): 111-117.

8) BORENSZTAJN, J., ET AL. (1970). "EFFECT OF FASTING ON THE CLEARING FACTOR LIPASE (LIPOPROTEIN LIPASE) ACTIVITY OF FRESH AND DEFATTED PREPARATIONS OF RAT HEART MUSCLE." J LIPID RES 11(2): 102-110.

9) TINSLEY, G. M., ET AL. (2017). "TIME-RESTRICTED FEEDING IN YOUNG MEN PERFORMING RESISTANCE TRAINING: A RANDOMIZED CONTROLLED TRIAL." EUR J SPORT SCI 17(2): 200-207.

10) LA BOUNTY, P. M., ET AL. (2011). "INTERNATIONAL SOCIETY OF SPORTS NUTRITION POSITION STAND: MEAL FREQUENCY." J INT SOC SPORTS NUTR 8: 4.

11) LEIDY, H. J. AND W. W. CAMPBELL (2011). "THE EFFECT OF EATING FREQUENCY ON APPETITE CONTROL AND FOOD INTAKE: BRIEF SYNOPSIS OF CONTROLLED FEEDING STUDIES." J NUTR 141(1): 154-157.

12) TINSLEY, G. M. AND P. M. LA BOUNTY (2015). "EFFECTS OF INTERMITTENT FASTING ON BODY COMPOSITION AND CLINICAL HEALTH MARKERS IN HUMANS." NUTR REV 73(10): 661-674.

13) ZUO, L., ET AL. (2016). "COMPARISON OF HIGH-PROTEIN, INTERMITTENT FASTING LOW-CALORIE DIET AND HEART HEALTHY DIET FOR VASCULAR HEALTH OF THE OBESE." FRONT PHYSIOL 7: 350.

14) BROOKS, G. A. AND J. MERCIER (1994). "BALANCE OF CARBOHYDRATE AND LIPID UTILIZATION DURING EXERCISE: THE "CROSSOVER" CONCEPT." J APPL PHYSIOL (1985) 76(6): 2253-2261.

15) BROOKS, G. A. (1987). "AMINO ACID AND PROTEIN METABOLISM DURING EXERCISE AND RECOVERY." MED SCI SPORTS EXERC 19(5 SUPPL): S150-156.

16) ROBERGS, R. A., ET AL. (1991). "MUSCLE GLYCOGENOLYSIS DURING DIFFERING INTENSITIES OF WEIGHT-RESISTANCE EXERCISE." J APPL PHYSIOL (1985) 70(4): 1700-1706.

17) FOURNIER, P. A., ET AL. (2004). "POST-EXERCISE MUSCLE GLYCOGEN REPLETION IN THE EXTREME: EFFECT OF FOOD ABSENCE AND ACTIVE RECOVERY." J SPORTS SCI MED 3(3): 139-146.

18) KERKSICK, C. M., ET AL. (2017). "INTERNATIONAL SOCIETY OF SPORTS NUTRITION POSITION STAND: NUTRIENT TIMING." J INT SOC SPORTS NUTR 14: 33.

19) ARAGON, A. A. AND B. J. SCHOENFELD (2013). "NUTRIENT TIMING REVISITED: IS THERE A POST-EXERCISE ANABOLIC WINDOW?" J INT SOC SPORTS NUTR 10(1): 5.

20) STARK, M., ET AL. (2012). "PROTEIN TIMING AND ITS EFFECTS ON MUSCULAR HYPERTROPHY AND STRENGTH IN INDIVIDUALS ENGAGED IN WEIGHT-TRAINING." J INT SOC SPORTS NUTR 9(1): 54.

21) PATEL, S. R. AND F. B. HU (2008). "SHORT SLEEP DURATION AND WEIGHT GAIN: A SYSTEMATIC REVIEW." OBESITY (SILVER SPRING) 16(3): 643-653.

22) NATIONAL RESEARCH COUNCIL (NRC). RECOMMENDED DIETARY ALLOWANCES, 10TH ED. WASHINGTON, DC: NATIONAL ACADEMY OF SCIENCES; 1989.

23) JAGER, R., ET AL. (2017). "INTERNATIONAL SOCIETY OF SPORTS NUTRITION POSITION STAND: PROTEIN AND EXERCISE." J INT SOC SPORTS NUTR 14: 20.

24) APPEL, L. J., ET AL. (2005). "EFFECTS OF PROTEIN, MONOUNSATURATED FAT, AND CARBOHYDRATE INTAKE ON BLOOD PRESSURE AND SERUM LIPIDS: RESULTS OF THE OMNIHEART RANDOMIZED TRIAL." JAMA 294(19): 2455-2464.

25) POORTMANS, J. R. AND O. DELLALIEUX (2000). "DO REGULAR HIGH PROTEIN DIETS HAVE POTENTIAL HEALTH RISKS ON KIDNEY FUNCTION IN ATHLETES?" INT J SPORT NUTR EXERC METAB 10(1): 28-38.

26) GINTY, F. (2003). "DIETARY PROTEIN AND BONE HEALTH." PROC NUTR SOC 62(4): 867-876.

27) RIZZOLI, R., ET AL. (2010). "MAXIMIZING BONE MINERAL MASS GAIN DURING GROWTH FOR THE PREVENTION OF FRACTURES IN THE ADOLESCENTS AND THE ELDERLY." BONE 46(2): 294-305.

28) NEW, S. A., ET AL. (2004). "LOWER ESTIMATES OF NET ENDOGENOUS NON-CARBONIC ACID PRODUCTION ARE POSITIVELY ASSOCIATED WITH INDEXES OF BONE HEALTH IN PREMENOPAUSAL AND PERIMENOPAUSAL WOMEN." AM J CLIN NUTR 79(1): 131-138.

29) ANTONIO, J., ET AL. (2014). "THE EFFECTS OF CONSUMING A HIGH PROTEIN DIET (4.4 G/KG/D) ON BODY COMPOSITION IN RESISTANCE-TRAINED INDIVIDUALS." J INT SOC SPORTS NUTR 11: 19.

30) ANTONIO, J., ET AL. (2015). "A HIGH PROTEIN DIET (3.4 G/KG/D) COMBINED WITH A HEAVY RESISTANCE TRAINING PROGRAM IMPROVES BODY COMPOSITION IN HEALTHY TRAINED MEN AND WOMEN--A FOLLOW-UP INVESTIGATION." J INT SOC SPORTS NUTR 12: 39.

31) WEIGLE, D. S., ET AL. (2005). "A HIGH-PROTEIN DIET INDUCES SUSTAINED REDUCTIONS IN APPETITE, AD LIBITUM CALORIC INTAKE, AND BODY WEIGHT DESPITE COMPENSATORY CHANGES IN DIURNAL PLASMA LEPTIN AND GHRELIN CONCENTRATIONS." AM J CLIN NUTR 82(1): 41-48.

32) ANTONIO, J., ET AL. (2016). "THE EFFECTS OF A HIGH PROTEIN DIET ON INDICES OF HEALTH AND BODY COMPOSITION--A CROSSOVER TRIAL IN RESISTANCE-TRAINED MEN." J INT SOC SPORTS NUTR 13: 3.

33) MORALES, F. E. M., ET AL. (2017). "ACUTE AND LONG-TERM IMPACT OF HIGH-PROTEIN DIETS ON ENDOCRINE AND METABOLIC FUNCTION, BODY COMPOSITION, AND EXERCISE-INDUCED ADAPTATIONS." J AM COLL NUTR 36(4): 295-305.

34) SCHOENFELD, B. J., ET AL. (2013). "THE EFFECT OF PROTEIN TIMING ON MUSCLE STRENGTH AND HYPERTROPHY: A META-ANALYSIS." J INT SOC SPORTS NUTR 10(1): 53.

35) STARK, M., ET AL. (2012). "PROTEIN TIMING AND ITS EFFECTS ON MUSCULAR HYPERTROPHY AND STRENGTH IN INDIVIDUALS ENGAGED IN WEIGHT-TRAINING." J INT SOC SPORTS NUTR 9(1): 54.

36) COOK, J. D., ET AL. (1994). "IRON DEFICIENCY: THE GLOBAL PERSPECTIVE." ADV EXP MED BIOL 356: 219-228.

37) PITTAS, A. G., ET AL. (2007). "THE ROLE OF VITAMIN D AND CALCIUM IN TYPE 2 DIABETES. A SYSTEMATIC REVIEW AND META-ANALYSIS." J CLIN ENDOCRINOL METAB 92(6): 2017-2029.

38) PALOMER, X., ET AL. (2008). "ROLE OF VITAMIN D IN THE PATHOGENESIS OF TYPE 2 DIABETES MELLITUS." DIABETES OBES METAB 10(3): 185-197.

39) GARNERO, P., ET AL. (2007). "ASSOCIATIONS OF VITAMIN D STATUS WITH BONE MINERAL DENSITY, BONE TURNOVER, BONE LOSS AND FRACTURE RISK IN HEALTHY POSTMENOPAUSAL WOMEN. THE OFELY STUDY." BONE 40(3): 716-722.

40) MITRI, J., ET AL. (2011). "EFFECTS OF VITAMIN D AND CALCIUM SUPPLEMENTATION ON PANCREATIC BETA CELL FUNCTION, INSULIN SENSITIVITY, AND GLYCEMIA IN ADULTS AT HIGH RISK OF DIABETES: THE CALCIUM AND VITAMIN D FOR DIABETES MELLITUS (CADDM) RANDOMIZED CONTROLLED TRIAL." AM J CLIN NUTR 94(2): 486-494.

41) SINGLA, M., ET AL. (2017). "VITAMIN D SUPPLEMENTATION IMPROVES SIMVASTATIN-MEDIATED DECLINE IN EXERCISE PERFORMANCE: A RANDOMIZED DOUBLE-BLIND PLACEBO-CONTROLLED STUDY." J DIABETES.

42) REID, I. R., ET AL. (2014). "EFFECTS OF VITAMIN D SUPPLEMENTS ON BONE MINERAL DENSITY: A SYSTEMATIC REVIEW AND META-ANALYSIS." LANCET 383(9912): 146-155.

43) O'HARA, A. M. AND F. SHANAHAN (2006). "THE GUT FLORA AS A FORGOTTEN ORGAN." EMBO REP 7(7): 688-693.

44) LUNDIN, A., ET AL. (2008). "GUT FLORA, TOLL-LIKE RECEPTORS AND NUCLEAR RECEPTORS: A TRIPARTITE COMMUNICATION THAT TUNES INNATE IMMUNITY IN LARGE INTESTINE." CELL MICROBIOL 10(5): 1093-1103.

45) JUMPERTZ, R., ET AL. (2011). "ENERGY-BALANCE STUDIES REVEAL ASSOCIATIONS BETWEEN GUT MICROBES, CALORIC LOAD, AND NUTRIENT ABSORPTION IN HUMANS." AM J CLIN NUTR 94(1): 58-65.

46) SHANAHAN, F. (2002). "THE HOST-MICROBE INTERFACE WITHIN THE GUT." BEST PRACT RES CLIN GASTROENTEROL 16(6): 915-931.

47) GRONLUND, M. M., ET AL. (1999). "FECAL MICROFLORA IN HEALTHY INFANTS BORN BY DIFFERENT METHODS OF DELIVERY: PERMANENT CHANGES IN INTESTINAL FLORA AFTER CESAREAN DELIVERY." J PEDIATR GASTROENTEROL NUTR 28(1): 19-25.

48) KIM, S., ET AL. (2017). "THE INTESTINAL MICROBIOTA: ANTIBIOTICS, COLONIZATION RESISTANCE, AND ENTERIC PATHOGENS." IMMUNOL REV 279(1): 90-105.

49) ZUBIRIA, M. G., ET AL. (2017). "DELETERIOUS METABOLIC EFFECTS OF HIGH FRUCTOSE INTAKE: THE PREVENTIVE EFFECT OF LACTOBACILLUS KEFIRI ADMINISTRATION." NUTRIENTS 9(5)

50) ISOLAURI, E., ET AL. (2001). "PROBIOTICS: EFFECTS ON IMMUNITY." AM J CLIN NUTR 73(2 SUPPL): 444S-450S.

51) MARETTI, C. AND G. CAVALLINI (2017). "THE ASSOCIATION OF A PROBIOTIC WITH A PREBIOTIC (FLORTEC, BRACCO) TO IMPROVE THE QUALITY/QUANTITY OF SPERMATOZOA IN INFERTILE PATIENTS WITH IDIOPATHIC OLIGOASTHENOTERATOSPERMIA: A PILOT STUDY." ANDROLOGY 5(3): 439-444.

52) FOOKS, L. J. AND G. R. GIBSON (2002). "PROBIOTICS AS MODULATORS OF THE GUT FLORA." BR J NUTR 88 SUPPL 1: S39-49.

53) WILLIAMS, B. A., ET AL. (2017). "GUT FERMENTATION OF DIETARY FIBRES: PHYSICO-CHEMISTRY OF PLANT CELL WALLS AND IMPLICATIONS FOR HEALTH." INT J MOL SCI 18(10).

54) MATSUSHITA, H., ET AL. (2008). "DIETARY FISH OIL RESULTS IN A GREATER BONE MASS AND BONE FORMATION INDICES IN AGED OVARIECTOMIZED RATS." J BONE MINER METAB 26(3): 241-247.

55) YOSHINO, J., ET AL. (2016). "EFFECT OF DIETARY N-3 PUFA SUPPLEMENTATION ON THE MUSCLE TRANSCRIPTOME IN OLDER ADULTS." PHYSIOL REP 4(11).

56) FABER, J., ET AL. (2011). "SUPPLEMENTATION WITH A FISH OIL-ENRICHED, HIGH-PROTEIN MEDICAL FOOD LEADS TO RAPID INCORPORATION OF EPA INTO WHITE BLOOD CELLS AND MODULATES IMMUNE RESPONSES WITHIN ONE WEEK IN HEALTHY MEN AND WOMEN." J NUTR 141(5): 964-970.

57) SHEN, J., ET AL. (2016). "OMEGA-3 FATTY ACID SUPPLEMENT PREVENTS DEVELOPMENT OF INTRACRANIAL ATHEROSCLEROSIS." NEUROSCIENCE 334: 226-235.

58) JOY, J. M., ET AL. (2013). "THE EFFECTS OF 8 WEEKS OF WHEY OR RICE PROTEIN SUPPLEMENTATION ON BODY COMPOSITION AND EXERCISE PERFORMANCE." NUTR J 12: 86.

59) HOFFMAN, J. R. AND M. J. FALVO (2004). "PROTEIN - WHICH IS BEST?" J SPORTS SCI MED 3(3): 118-130.

60) TROCK, B. J., ET AL. (2006). "META-ANALYSIS OF SOY INTAKE AND BREAST CANCER RISK." J NATL CANCER INST 98(7): 459-471.

61) CHEN, M., ET AL. (2014). "ASSOCIATION BETWEEN SOY ISOFLAVONE INTAKE AND BREAST CANCER RISK FOR PRE- AND POST-MENOPAUSAL WOMEN: A META-ANALYSIS OF EPIDEMIOLOGICAL STUDIES." PLOS ONE 9(2): E89288.

62) HAMILTON-REEVES, J. M., ET AL. (2010). "CLINICAL STUDIES SHOW NO EFFECTS OF SOY PROTEIN OR ISOFLAVONES ON REPRODUCTIVE HORMONES IN MEN: RESULTS OF A META-ANALYSIS." FERTIL STERIL 94(3): 997-1007.

63) BOIRIE, Y., ET AL. (1997). "SLOW AND FAST DIETARY PROTEINS DIFFERENTLY MODULATE POSTPRANDIAL PROTEIN ACCRETION." PROC NATL ACAD SCI U S A 94(26): 14930-14935.

64) TIPTON, K. D., ET AL. (2004). "INGESTION OF CASEIN AND WHEY PROTEINS RESULT IN MUSCLE ANABOLISM AFTER RESISTANCE EXERCISE." MED SCI SPORTS EXERC 36(12): 2073-2081.

65) GEISER, M. (2003). "THE WONDERS OF WHEY PROTEIN." NSCA'S PERFORMANCE TRAINING JOURNAL 2, 13-15.

66) PADDON-JONES, D., ET AL. (2004). "AMINO ACID INGESTION IMPROVES MUSCLE PROTEIN SYNTHESIS IN THE YOUNG AND ELDERLY." AM J PHYSIOL ENDOCRINOL METAB, 286:E321–E328.

67) TIPTON K., ET AL. (1999). "POSTEXERCISE NET PROTEIN SYNTHESIS IN HUMAN MUSCLE FROM ORALLY ADMINISTERED AMINO ACIDS." AM J PHYSIOL, 276:E628–E634.

68) TIPTON, K. D., ET AL. (2001). "TIMING OF AMINO ACID-CARBOHYDRATE INGESTION ALTERS ANABOLIC RESPONSE OF MUSCLE TO RESISTANCE EXERCISE." AM J PHYSIOL ENDOCRINOL METAB, 281:E197-E206.

69) CHURCHWARD-VENNE, T. A., ET AL. (2014). "LEUCINE SUPPLEMENTATION OF A LOW-PROTEIN MIXED MACRONUTRIENT BEVERAGE ENHANCES MYOFIBRILLAR PROTEIN SYNTHESIS IN YOUNG MEN: A DOUBLE-BLIND, RANDOMIZED TRIAL." AM J CLIN NUTR 99(2): 276-286.

70) JONKER, R., ET AL. (2017). "EFFECTIVENESS OF ESSENTIAL AMINO ACID SUPPLEMENTATION IN STIMULATING WHOLE BODY NET PROTEIN ANABOLISM IS COMPARABLE BETWEEN COPD PATIENTS AND HEALTHY OLDER ADULTS." METABOLISM 69: 120-129.

71) BORSHEIM, E., ET AL. (2002). "ESSENTIAL AMINO ACIDS AND MUSCLE PROTEIN RECOVERY FROM RESISTANCE EXERCISE." AM J PHYSIOL ENDOCRINOL METAB 283(4): E648-657.

72) BROSNAN, M. E. AND J. T. BROSNAN (2016). "THE ROLE OF DIETARY CREATINE." AMINO ACIDS 48(8): 1785-1791.

73) PADDON-JONES, D., ET AL. (2004). "POTENTIAL ERGOGENIC EFFECTS OF ARGININE AND CREATINE SUPPLEMENTATION." J NUTR 134(10 SUPPL): 2888S-2894S; DISCUSSION 2895S.

74) HULTMAN, E., ET AL. (1996). "MUSCLE CREATINE LOADING IN MEN." J APPL PHYSIOL (1985) 81(1): 232-237.

75) KREIDER, R. B., ET AL. (2017). "INTERNATIONAL SOCIETY OF SPORTS NUTRITION POSITION STAND: SAFETY AND EFFICACY OF CREATINE SUPPLEMENTATION IN EXERCISE, SPORT, AND MEDICINE." J INT SOC SPORTS NUTR 14: 18.

76) BUFORD, T. W., ET AL. (2007). "INTERNATIONAL SOCIETY OF SPORTS NUTRITION POSITION STAND: CREATINE SUPPLEMENTATION AND EXERCISE." J INT SOC SPORTS NUTR 4: 6.

77) NADERI, A., ET AL. (2016). "TIMING, OPTIMAL DOSE AND INTAKE DURATION OF DIETARY SUPPLEMENTS WITH EVIDENCE-BASED USE IN SPORTS NUTRITION." J EXERC NUTRITION BIOCHEM 20(4): 1-12.

78) POORTMANS, J. R. AND M. FRANCAUX (2000). "ADVERSE EFFECTS OF CREATINE SUPPLEMENTATION: FACT OR FICTION?" SPORTS MED 30(3): 155-170.

79) KILDUFF LP, ET AL. "THE EFFECTS OF CREATINE SUPPLEMENTATION ON CARDIOVASCULAR, METABOLIC, AND THERMOREGULATORY RESPONSES DURING EXERCISE IN THE HEAT IN ENDURANCE-TRAINED HUMANS." INT J SPORT NUTR EXERC METAB. 2004;14(4):443–60.

80) WATSON G, ET AL. "CREATINE USE AND EXERCISE HEAT TOLERANCE IN DEHYDRATED MEN." J ATHL TRAIN. 2006;41(1):18–29.

81) TREXLER, E. T., ET AL. (2015). "INTERNATIONAL SOCIETY OF SPORTS NUTRITION POSITION STAND: BETA-ALANINE." J INT SOC SPORTS NUTR 12: 30.

82) MONCADA, S. AND A. HIGGS (1993). "THE L-ARGININE-NITRIC OXIDE PATHWAY." N ENGL J MED 329(27): 2002-2012.

83) PALMER, R. M., ET AL. (1988). "L-ARGININE IS THE PHYSIOLOGICAL PRECURSOR FOR THE FORMATION OF NITRIC OXIDE IN ENDOTHELIUM-DEPENDENT RELAXATION." BIOCHEM BIOPHYS RES COMMUN 153(3): 1251-1256.

84) AGARWAL, U., ET AL. (2017). "SUPPLEMENTAL CITRULLINE IS MORE EFFICIENT THAN ARGININE IN INCREASING SYSTEMIC ARGININE AVAILABILITY IN MICE." J NUTR 147(4): 596-602.

85) BAILEY, S. J., ET AL. (2015). "L-CITRULLINE SUPPLEMENTATION IMPROVES O2 UPTAKE KINETICS AND HIGH-INTENSITY EXERCISE PERFORMANCE IN HUMANS." J APPL PHYSIOL (1985) 119(4): 385-395.

86) TREXLER, E. T., ET AL. (2019). "ACUTE EFFECTS OF CITRULLINE SUPPLEMENTATION ON HIGH-INTENSITY STRENGTH AND POWER PERFORMANCE: A SYSTEMATIC REVIEW AND META-ANALYSIS." SPORTS MED 49(5): 707-718.

87) MEADOR, K. J., ET AL. (1993). "EVIDENCE FOR A CENTRAL CHOLINERGIC EFFECT OF HIGH-DOSE THIAMINE." ANN NEUROL 34(5): 724-726.

88) WEIGHT, L. M., ET AL. (1988). "VITAMIN AND MINERAL STATUS OF TRAINED ATHLETES INCLUDING THE EFFECTS OF SUPPLEMENTATION." AM J CLIN NUTR 47(2): 186-191.

89) GOLDSTEIN, E. R., ET AL. (2010). "INTERNATIONAL SOCIETY OF SPORTS NUTRITION POSITION STAND: CAFFEINE AND PERFORMANCE." J INT SOC SPORTS NUTR 7(1): 5.

90) SPRIET, L. L. (1995). "CAFFEINE AND PERFORMANCE." INT J SPORT NUTR 5 SUPPL: S84-99.

91) SPRIET, L. L., ET AL. (1992). "CAFFEINE INGESTION AND MUSCLE METABOLISM DURING PROLONGED EXERCISE IN HUMANS." AM J PHYSIOL 262(6 PT 1): E891-898.

92) LAURENT, D., ET AL. (2000). "EFFECTS OF CAFFEINE ON MUSCLE GLYCOGEN UTILIZATION AND THE NEUROENDOCRINE AXIS DURING EXERCISE." J CLIN ENDOCRINOL METAB 85(6): 2170-2175.

93) GROSSMAN, A. AND J. R. SUTTON (1985). "ENDORPHINS: WHAT ARE THEY? HOW ARE THEY MEASURED? WHAT IS THEIR ROLE IN EXERCISE?" MED SCI SPORTS EXERC 17(1): 74-81.

94) LOPES, J. M., ET AL. (1983). "EFFECT OF CAFFEINE ON SKELETAL MUSCLE FUNCTION BEFORE AND AFTER FATIGUE." J APPL PHYSIOL RESPIR ENVIRON EXERC PHYSIOL 54(5): 1303-1305.

95) HOFFMAN, J. R., ET AL. (2009). "POSITION STAND ON ANDROGEN AND HUMAN GROWTH HORMONE USE." J STRENGTH COND RES 23(5 SUPPL): S1-S59.

96) MAURAS, N., ET AL. (2003). "SYNERGISTIC EFFECTS OF TESTOSTERONE AND GROWTH HORMONE ON PROTEIN METABOLISM AND BODY COMPOSITION IN PREPUBERTAL BOYS." METABOLISM 52(8): 964-969.

97) BLEISCH, W., ET AL. (1984). "MODIFICATION OF SYNAPSES IN ANDROGEN-SENSITIVE MUSCLE. I. HORMONAL REGULATION OF ACETYLCHOLINE RECEPTOR NUMBER IN THE SONGBIRD SYRINX." J NEUROSCI 4(3): 786-792.

98) BHASIN, S., ET AL. (1996). "THE EFFECTS OF SUPRAPHYSIOLOGIC DOSES OF TESTOSTERONE ON MUSCLE SIZE AND STRENGTH IN NORMAL MEN." N ENGL J MED 335(1): 1-7.

99) HYLDAHL, R. D., ET AL. (2014). "SATELLITE CELL ACTIVITY IS DIFFERENTIALLY AFFECTED BY CONTRACTION MODE IN HUMAN MUSCLE FOLLOWING A WORK-MATCHED BOUT OF EXERCISE." FRONT PHYSIOL 5: 485.

100) SINHA-HIKIM, I., ET AL. (2003). "TESTOSTERONE-INDUCED MUSCLE HYPERTROPHY IS ASSOCIATED WITH AN INCREASE IN SATELLITE CELL NUMBER IN HEALTHY, YOUNG MEN." AM J PHYSIOL ENDOCRINOL METAB 285(1): E197-205.

101) WALSH, F. S. AND A. J. CELESTE (2005). "MYOSTATIN: A MODULATOR OF SKELETAL-MUSCLE STEM CELLS." BIOCHEM SOC TRANS 33(PT 6): 1513-1517. 5)

102) MENDLER, L., ET AL. (2007). "ANDROGENS NEGATIVELY REGULATE MYOSTATIN EXPRESSION IN AN ANDROGEN-DEPENDENT SKELETAL MUSCLE." BIOCHEM BIOPHYS RES COMMUN 361(1): 237-242.

103) SINHA-HIKIM, I., ET AL. (2006). "EFFECTS OF TESTOSTERONE SUPPLEMENTATION ON SKELETAL MUSCLE FIBER HYPERTROPHY AND SATELLITE CELLS IN COMMUNITY-DWELLING OLDER MEN." J CLIN ENDOCRINOL METAB 91(8): 3024-3033.

104) CORONA, G., ET AL. (2014). "TESTOSTERONE SUPPLEMENTATION AND SEXUAL FUNCTION: A META-ANALYSIS STUDY." J SEX MED 11(6): 1577-1592.

105) HAFEZ, B. AND E. S. HAFEZ (2004). "ANDROPAUSE: ENDOCRINOLOGY, ERECTILE DYSFUNCTION, AND PROSTATE PATHOPHYSIOLOGY." ARCH ANDROL 50(2): 45-68.

106) BHASIN, S. (2003). "EFFECTS OF TESTOSTERONE ADMINISTRATION ON FAT DISTRIBUTION, INSULIN SENSITIVITY, AND ATHEROSCLEROSIS PROGRESSION." CLIN INFECT DIS 37 SUPPL 2: S142-149.

107) SCHWARZ, S., ET AL. (1999). "THE STEROID STORY OF JENAPHARM: FROM THE LATE 1940S TO THE EARLY 1970S." STEROIDS 64(7): 439-445.

108) TRICKER, R., ET AL. (1996). "THE EFFECTS OF SUPRAPHYSIOLOGICAL DOSES OF TESTOSTERONE ON ANGRY BEHAVIOR IN HEALTHY EUGONADAL MEN--A CLINICAL RESEARCH CENTER STUDY." J CLIN ENDOCRINOL METAB 81(10): 3754-3758.

109) LAKSHMAN, K. M., ET AL. (2010). "THE EFFECTS OF INJECTED TESTOSTERONE DOSE AND AGE ON THE CONVERSION OF TESTOSTERONE TO ESTRADIOL AND DIHYDROTESTOSTERONE IN YOUNG AND OLDER MEN." J CLIN ENDOCRINOL METAB 95(8): 3955-3964.

110) KREIDER, R. B., ET AL. (2010). "ISSN EXERCISE & SPORT NUTRITION REVIEW: RESEARCH & RECOMMENDATIONS." J INT SOC SPORTS NUTR 7: 7.

111) TINSLEY, G. M., ET AL. (2017). "EFFECTS OF TWO PRE-WORKOUT SUPPLEMENTS ON CONCENTRIC AND ECCENTRIC FORCE PRODUCTION DURING LOWER BODY RESISTANCE EXERCISE IN MALES AND FEMALES: A COUNTERBALANCED, DOUBLE-BLIND, PLACEBO-CONTROLLED TRIAL." J INT SOC SPORTS NUTR 14: 46.